Experts' Perspectives on Medical Advances

This book series presents Chinese experts' perspectives on recent developments in clinical medicine. Written by leading Chinese experts in related fields, a wide variety of emerging and hot topics in internal medicine, surgery, oncology, neurosurgery, and ophthalmonology, etc., is covered by the series. Each title in this series covers a disease or a group of diseases, focusing on the basic knowledge, development and the latest research progress of clinical practice. This series is a practical and useful resource for researchers and practitioners in related subjects, as well as for general interest readers.

Qing Zhou • Jian Chen

Ocular Myasthenia Gravis

Springer

科学技术文献出版社
SCIENTIFIC AND TECHNICAL DOCUMENTATION PRESS

Qing Zhou
Department of Ophthalmology
First Affiliated Hospital of Jinan
University
Guangzhou, China

Jian Chen
Department of Ophthalmology
First Affiliated Hospital of Jinan
University
Guangzhou, China

ISSN 2948-1023 ISSN 2948-1031 (electronic)
Experts' Perspectives on Medical Advances
ISBN 978-981-96-1244-4 ISBN 978-981-96-1245-1 (eBook)
https://doi.org/10.1007/978-981-96-1245-1

The original submitted manuscript has been translated into English. The translation was done using artificial intelligence. A subsequent revision was performed by the author(s) to further refine the work and to ensure that the translation is appropriate concerning content and scientific correctness. It may, however, read stylistically different from a conventional translation.

Translation from the Chinese language edition: "眼肌型重症肌无力周清2022观点" by Qing Zhou and Jian Chen, © Scientific and Technical Documentation Press Co., Ltd. 2022. Published by Scientific and Technical Documentation Press Co., Ltd.. All Rights Reserved.

Jointly published with Scientific and Technical Documentation Press

This Springer imprint is published by the registered company Springer Nature Singapore Pte Ltd.
The registered company address is: 152 Beach Road, #21-01/04 Gateway East, Singapore 189721, Singapore

Preface

Myasthenia gravis (MG) is an autoimmune disease characterized by the production of autoantibodies that affect the neuromuscular junction, causing neuromuscular transmission disorders and resulting in muscle weakness. The antibodies produced include acetylcholine receptor antibodies, muscle-specific tyrosine kinase receptor antibodies, and low-density lipoprotein receptor-related protein 4 antibodies, etc. The typical symptom of myasthenia gravis is fluctuating muscle fatigue. MG is divided into ocular myasthenia gravis (OMG) and generalized myasthenia gravis (GMG). Ptosis, diplopia, and incomplete eyelid closure are usually the initial symptoms of MG, which can progress to affect other muscle groups, including respiratory muscles, leading to life-threatening situations. MG can have acute or subacute attacks (more common), with symptoms fluctuating and potential for recurrence and remission.

OMG is a type of MG that only involves the extraocular muscles, levator palpebrae superioris, and orbicularis oculi, accounting for about half of all MG patients. If not diagnosed and treated in time, it can severely affect the patient's quality of life and even cause disability. Early diagnosis and treatment are key to improving the patient's quality of life and reducing the transformation of OMG to GMG. However, the misdiagnosis rate of OMG is as high as 40%. Firstly, the clinical manifestations of OMG are diverse, and early symptoms are similar to other diseases, often misdiagnosed as thyroid-related eye disease, oculomotor nerve paralysis, or motor neuron disease. Secondly, early fluctuating, fatigue-prone ocular muscle weakness, which is relieved after rest, is an important basis for the clinical diagnosis of ocular myasthenia gravis. However, patients often fail to seek medical treatment in time due to mild early symptoms, and often seek medical treatment only when obvious ptosis or diplopia significantly affects normal life, increasing the difficulty of diagnosis. In addition, the low positivity rate of serum antibodies and electromyography is also a major cause of misdiagnosis. The purpose of OMG treatment is to relieve eye symptoms and delay or prevent the progression of OMG to GMG. The current treatment of OMG is not effective for refractory patients. Therefore, there are still many challenges in the diagnosis and treatment of OMG. This book mainly introduces ocular myasthenia gravis from the aspects of epidemiology, etiology and inducement, pathogenesis, clinical features, auxiliary examination, diagnosis and differential diagnosis, and treatment, as a reference book for guiding the diagnosis, treatment, and prognosis of OMG in clinical practice.

Finally, I would like to express my heartfelt thanks to my doctoral student, Dr. Yuanting Yang, who has spent a lot of time and effort in literature review and drafting the initial manuscript! At the same time, I would like to express my sincere thanks to the editors and staff of the Science and Technology Literature Publishing House and Springer Publishing House!

Guangzhou, China Qing Zhou

Contents

About the Authors

Qing Zhou Currently serving as the Director of the Department of Ophthalmology at the First Clinical Medical College of Jinan University, Executive Deputy Director of the Department of Ophthalmology at the First Affiliated Hospital of Jinan University. Youth Committee Member of the Ophthalmology Branch of the Chinese Medical Association, Committee Member of the Ophthalmic Tumor Special Committee of the Ophthalmology Branch of the Chinese Medical Association, Standing Committee Member of the Ophthalmology Branch of the Guangdong Medical Association, Deputy Group Leader of the Optometry and Amblyopia Professional Group of the Ophthalmology Branch of the Guangdong Medical Association, Deputy Director of the Ophthalmology Branch of the Guangzhou Medical Association, etc. Serving as a Corresponding Editorial Board Member of the *Chinese Journal of Optometry Ophthalmology and Visual Science*, and an Editorial Board Member of the *Journal of Wenzhou Medical University*, *Journal of Jinan University Medical Edition*, and *Guangdong Medicine*. Peer review expert of the National Natural Science Foundation of China.

Engaged in ophthalmology for 30 years, proficient in strabismus correction surgery, excimer laser myopia correction surgery, cataract phacoemulsification surgery, eye tumor and eye plastic surgery, and the diagnosis and treatment of difficult ophthalmic diseases such as ocular myasthenia gravis. In 2018, she was awarded the title of "Outstanding Young and Middle-aged Doctor of Guangdong Province," in 2019, she was awarded the title of "Lingnan Famous Doctor," and in 2020, she was awarded the title of "Good Doctor in Yangcheng." In scientific research, she has been engaged in the research of eye tissue regeneration, the application of stem cells in eye tissues, and ocular myasthenia gravis. She has presided over two projects of the National Natural Science Foundation of China; more than 10 provincial, municipal, and school-level scientific research fund projects; published more than 90 papers in domestic and foreign journals (including corresponding authors of papers in SCI including Biomater Adv, Stem Cell Res, Exp Eye Res, Expert Opin Ther Targets, J Tissue Eng Regen Med, etc.). She is the chief editor of *Ocular Myasthenia Gravis Zhou Qing 2022 Viewpoint*. Participated in the compilation of the fourth edition of the *Ophthalmology* of the *Fourteenth Five-Year Plan* textbook of the National Health Commission, including two copies of the paper version and the digital version. Participated in the compilation of the People's Health Publishing House's *National Advanced Health Professional Qualification Examination Guide Ophthalmology*, *National Advanced Health Professional Qualification*

Examination Exercise Set Series Ophthalmology Exercise Set, *Q&A on Ocular Tumor-Related Knowledge*, *Ophthalmology Learning Question Set* and other works, as well as the compilation of *Basic Theory and Clinical Practice of Ocular Surface Diseases* and *Chinese and Western Corneal Disease Studies*. Authorized two patents. As a major participant, she won the Guangdong Provincial Science and Technology Progress Second Prize twice in 2003 and 2005. In 2004, she won the Excellent Paper Award of the National Optometry Academic Symposium. In 2009, she was awarded the "Outstanding Contribution Award for Female Ophthalmologists in Guangdong Province" by the Guangdong Medical Association. In 2014, she won the Excellent Paper Award of the Guangdong Ophthalmology Annual Meeting. In 2022, she won the Second Prize of the Academic Exchange Competition of the Guangdong Ophthalmology Annual Meeting. From 2010 to the present, she has trained nearly 20 ophthalmology master's students and 6 doctoral students, and 2 postdoctoral fellows in the station.

Jian Chen Party Secretary of the School of Basic Medical Sciences and Public Health, Jinan University.

Having been engaged in medical education, research, and management for over 30 years, he was one of the first in China to carry out research on corneal limbal transplantation and amniotic membrane transplantation. He has successively served as a member of the Corneal Disease Group of the Ophthalmology Branch of the Chinese Medical Association; a member of the National Ocular Surface Disease Research Group; a member of the Eye Bank Collaboration Group; a national committee member of the Ophthalmology Branch of the Chinese Medical Association; a national committee member of the Ophthalmology Branch of the Chinese Medical Association; a national committee member of the Ophthalmology Branch of the Chinese Medical Equipment Association; vice chairman of the Ophthalmology Branch of the Guangdong Medical Association; vice chairman of the Humanities Medical Work Committee of the Guangdong Medical Association; and an editorial board member of the journals *Advances in Ophthalmology*, *Chinese Journal of Practical Ophthalmology*, *Ophthalmology Research*, and *Chinese Journal of Ophthalmology*. The series of studies on *Pathological Mechanism and Treatment of Ocular Alkali Burns* and *Basic and Clinical Studies on Ocular Surface Disease and Ocular Surface Reconstruction* that he led were awarded the second prize of Guangdong Province Science and Technology. In recent years, he has led and participated in more than 10 national, provincial, and municipal scientific research projects. He has contributed to the compilation of academic works and planned textbooks such as *Basics and Clinical Practice of Corneal Diseases*, *Basics and Clinical Practice of Ocular Surface Diseases*, *Integration of Traditional Chinese and Western Medicine in Corneal Diseases*, *Practical Ocular Surface Disease*, and *Geriatric Medicine*. He has published over 100 professional academic papers domestically and internationally. He has been awarded titles such as "Famous Doctor of Lingnan" and "Influential Doctor in China."

Overview and Epidemiology of Ocular Myasthenia Gravis

1

1.1 Brief History of Understanding Myasthenia Gravis

More than 300 years ago, human understanding of myasthenia gravis (MG) was very limited. It was not until 1672 that Thomas Willis [1] first detailed the manifestations of MG patients, including bulbar and truncal muscle weakness and the phenomenon of morning light and evening heavy, these symptoms are collectively referred to as "pseudoparalysis." Willis proposed that this weakness might be caused by fluctuations in the content of some "explosive medium" substance in the blood. Entering the nineteenth century, Erb [2] provided a more comprehensive description of MG, including symptoms such as bilateral ptosis and diplopia, and it was noted that some cases had temporary relief. In 1952, Dr. Goldflam [3] from Warsaw, Poland, analyzed the symptoms and prognosis of MG in detail and proposed differentiation from bulbar palsy and hysteria. He pointed out that MG patients have normal swallowing reflexes, no muscle atrophy and tremors, normal sphincter function, normal reflexes; but fatigue appears after repeated stimulation. Goldflam's paper is considered the "most important discourse in the history of MG understanding." Therefore, MG was once named Erb-Goldflam symptom-complex. In 1895, German physician Friedrich Jolly [4] proposed the term "myasthenia gravis" at a meeting of the Berlin Society, derived from Greek and Latin, meaning severe muscle weakness. Jolly also observed the phenomenon of gradually weakening muscle responsiveness in electrotherapy, which later developed into an important diagnostic method for myasthenia gravis—repetitive nerve stimulation (RNS) examination.

At the beginning of the twentieth century, the medical community began to pay attention to the connection between MG and the thymus. In 1911, Sauerbruch performed the first thymectomy on an MG patient in Zurich, Switzerland, and the patient's symptoms significantly improved after the operation. Since then, thymectomy has become an important means of treating MG. In 1934, Mary Walker [5] reported the transient effect of Physostigmine on MG, which was called the "St Alfege miracle." Later that year, she reported the significant effect of Neostigmine in the treatment of MG, opening a new path for the drug treatment of MG. By the mid-twentieth century, with a deeper understanding of the autoimmune mechanism of MG, corticosteroids and immunosuppressants began to be used in the treatment of MG. In addition, immunosuppressive biological agents such as cyclosporine and mycophenolate mofetil also showed effects in treatment. Plasma exchange and high-dose intravenous immunoglobulin (intravenous immunoglobulin, IVIG) as supportive treatments, provide new treatment options for MG patients.

Q. Zhou, J. Chen, *Ocular Myasthenia Gravis*, Experts' Perspectives on Medical Advances,
https://doi.org/10.1007/978-981-96-1245-1_1

In 1959–1960, Simpson and Nastuck proposed the autoimmune disease theory of MG [6, 7], and then in 1973, Patrick and Lindstrom's research showed that the acetylcholine receptor (AChR) is the target of autoimmune attack [8]. In 2001, Angela Carmen Vincent discovered the muscle-specific tyrosine kinase antibody (MuSK-Ab), further expanding the understanding of the autoimmune mechanism of MG, providing a new perspective for the pathogenesis and diagnosis of MG [9].

Over time, the clinical classification of MG has also been continuously developed. In 1958, Osserman first proposed the clinical classification of MG, and revised it in 1971, that is, the modified Osserman classification [10]. Osserman classified adult myasthenia gravis into five types, including I: Ocular; IIA: Mild generalized; IIB: Moderate generalized; III: Acute severe; IV: Late severe; V: Muscular atrophy. For over half a century, Osserman's classification has become the international standard for MG, widely adopted in clinical practice and is of significant importance for the study, treatment, and prognosis of MG. As our understanding of MG deepens, people have gradually discovered the shortcomings of Osserman's classification. The Myasthenia Gravis Foundation of America (MGFA) introduced the MGFA clinical classification and Quantitative MG score (QMG) based on quantitative testing in 2000, providing more precise tools for the diagnosis and treatment of MG [11]. These advancements have not only deepened our understanding of MG but also brought more effective evaluation methods for patients.

1.2 Ocular Myasthenia Gravis Is a Subtype of Myasthenia Gravis

Myasthenia gravis (MG) is an autoimmune disease characterized by fluctuating and fatigable skeletal muscle weakness, involving the postsynaptic membrane of the neuromuscular junction (NMJ) mediated by antibodies, cytokine-dependent, and complement-involved. These autoantibodies include acetylcholine receptors antibody (AChR-Ab), muscle-specific tyrosine kinase antibody (MuSK-Ab), and low-density lipoprotein receptor-related protein 4 antibody (LRP4-Ab), etc. Through a series of different pathogenic mechanisms, they alter the tissue architecture and the density or function of AChR, hinder neuromuscular transmission, thereby causing myasthenic symptoms. OMG is a type of MG that only involves the levator palpebrae superioris, extraocular muscles, and orbicularis oculi muscles, presenting symptoms such as ptosis, diplopia, strabismus, and incomplete eyelid closure. OMG is often missed and misdiagnosed due to its fluctuating symptoms, often leading to severe binocular visual impairment due to delayed treatment, causing serious harm to the quality of life as the disease progresses.

1.3 Ocular Myasthenia Gravis Accounts for About Half of Myasthenia Gravis

A study published in 2019 showed that the total incidence of MG is 2.2/100,000, the incidence of OMG is 1.13/100,000, and OMG accounts for about 51% of all MG patients [12]. The typical symptoms of OMG are ptosis and diplopia, which are the initial complaints of more than two-thirds of MG patients, and about 28% of OMG patients will transition to GMG in 2 years [13], similar to previous data from Asians in northwest China, southern China, Hong Kong, Korea, and Singapore (11.4%–29%) [14–18]. The incidence of MG in China is about 0.68/100,000, with a slightly higher incidence in women [19].

In China, statistics for the MG patient population show that the prevalence of MG in children and adolescents is as high as 50%, constituting the third peak of incidence; adolescent MG is mainly ocular, rarely transforming into generalized type [20]. The latest epidemiological survey shows that the age group of 70–74 years old is the high-risk population in our country [20].

References

1. Hughes JT. Thomas Willis (1621–1675). J Neurol. 2000;247(2):151–2. https://doi.org/10.1007/pl00007800.
2. Haymaker W, Schiller F. The founders of neurology. 2nd ed. Illinois: Charles C Thomas; 1970.
3. Herman E. Centenary of birth of Dr. Samuel Goldflam. Pol Tyg Lek. 1952;7:493–5.
4. Jolly F. Ueber myasthenia gravis pseudoparalytica. Berlin Klin Wochenschr. 1895;32:1–7.
5. Walker M. Treatment of myasthenia gravis with physostigmine. Lancet. 1934;1:1200–1.
6. Nastuk WL, Strauss AJ, et al. Search for a neuromuscular blocking agent in the blood of patients with myasuenla gravis. AmJ Med. 1959;26:194–409.
7. Simpson JA. Myasthenia gravis, a new hypohesis. Scott Med J. 1960;5:419–36.
8. Patrick J, Lindstrom J. Autoimmune response to acetylcholine receptor. Science. 1973;180(4088):871–2. https://doi.org/10.1126/science.180.4088.871.
9. Hoch W, McConville J, Helms S, et al. Autoantibodies to the receptor tyrosine kinase MuSK in patients with myasthenia gravis without acetylcholine receptor antibodies. Nat Med. 2001;7(3):365–8. https://doi.org/10.1038/85520.
10. Osserman KE, Genkins G. Studies in myasthenia gravis: review of a twenty-year experience in over 1200 patients. Mt Sinai J Med. 1971;38(6):497–537.
11. Jaretzki A 3rd, Barohn RJ, Ernstoff RM, et al. Myasthenia gravis: recommendations for clinical research standards. Task Force of the Medical Scientific Advisory Board of the Myasthenia Gravis Foundation of America. Ann Thorac Surg. 2000;70(1):327–34. https://doi.org/10.1016/s0003-4975(00)01595-2.
12. Kerty E, Elsais A, Argov Z, et al. EFNS/ENS Guidelines for the treatment of ocular myasthenia. Eur J Neurol. 2014;21(5):687–93. https://doi.org/10.1111/ene.12359.
13. Hendricks T, Bhatti M, Hodge D, et al. Incidence, epidemiology, and transformation of ocular myasthenia gravis: a population-based study. Am J Ophthalmol. 2019;205:99–105. https://doi.org/10.1016/j.ajo.2019.04.017.
14. Ding JQ, Zhao SJ, Ren KX, et al. Prediction of generalization of ocular myasthenia gravis under immunosuppressive therapy in Northwest China. BMC Neurol. 2020;20(1) https://doi.org/10.1186/s12883-020-01805-1.
15. Wang LL, Zhang Y, He ML. Clinical features and prognosis of ocular myasthenia gravis patients with different phenotypes. Chin Med J. 2015;128(19):2682–4. https://doi.org/10.4103/0366-6999.166032.
16. Kamarajah SK, Sadalage G, Palmer J, et al. Ocular presentation of myasthenia gravis: a natural history cohort. Muscle Nerve. 2018;57(4):622–7. https://doi.org/10.1002/mus.25971.
17. Nagia L, Lemos J, Abusamra K, et al. Prognosis of ocular myasthenia gravis retrospective multicenter analysis. Ophthalmology. 2015;122(7):1517–21. https://doi.org/10.1016/j.ophtha.2015.03.010.
18. Teo KY, Tow SL, Haaland B, et al. Low conversion rate of ocular to generalized myasthenia gravis in Singapore. Muscle Nerve. 2018;57(5):756–60. https://doi.org/10.1002/mus.25983.
19. Chen J, Tian D-C, Zhang C, et al. Incidence, mortality, and economic burden of myasthenia gravis in China: a nationwide population-based study. Lancet Reg Health West Pac. 2020;5:100063. https://doi.org/10.1016/j.lanwpc.2020.100063.
20. Huang X, Li Y, Feng H, et al. Clinical characteristics of juvenile myasthenia gravis in southern China. Front Neurol. 2018;9:77. https://doi.org/10.3389/fneur.2018.00077.

Pathophysiology of Ocular Myasthenia Gravis

2

2.1 The Pathophysiological Mechanism of OMG Is Related to the Destruction of the Normal Structure and Function of NMJ

The neuromuscular junction (NMJ) is the site responsible for impulse transmission between nerve endings and muscle fibers. This process requires the release of acetylcholine (ACh) from the presynaptic membrane and its binding to the acetylcholine receptor (AChR) on the postsynaptic membrane. Under normal physiological conditions, when the action potential reaches the motor nerve endings, the voltage-gated calcium ion channels are activated, causing calcium ions to flow into the nerve endings. Subsequently, synaptic vesicles containing ACh are released from the presynaptic membrane [1]. The spontaneous release of synaptic vesicles produces miniature end-plate potentials (mEPPs). During nerve impulses, the synchronous release of many synaptic vesicles leads to a large-scale depolarization of the end-plate membrane, and the addition of miniature end-plate potentials produces end-plate potentials (EPPs). When the peak of Epps reaches the critical threshold, it will trigger the action potential (AP) in the muscle fibers. In normal muscles, this series of events will occur in each nerve impulse. The binding of ACh to the receptor on the postsynaptic membrane opens the ACh cation-specific channel, causing local depolarization and activating adjacent voltage-gated sodium channels. This process converts chemical signals into electrical signals, i.e., the AP of muscle fibers. The role of acetylcholinesterase in the hydrolysis of ACh is crucial, which can prevent a single ACh molecule from repeatedly activating AChR. The effective nerve transmission of the neuromuscular junction originates from the amount of ACh released into the synapse being higher than the amount required to trigger the AP, thus maintaining long-term repetitive muscle fiber contraction [1, 2]. The part of the EPPs amplitude that exceeds the amplitude required to trigger the AP is called the "safety factor" [3]. The term "safety factor" is used to describe the effectiveness of NMJ transmission, specifically defined as the ratio between the actual neurotransmitter release produced by the nerve and the amount of neurotransmitter required to trigger the AP [3]. Factors affecting the safety factor of NMJ include the amount of ACh release, the density of AChR at the postsynaptic membrane and secondary postsynaptic membrane folds, and the density of sodium ion channels [2]. The density of AChR and sodium ion channels at the postsynaptic membrane folds depends on the presence of postsynaptic membrane folds, which determine the density of voltage-gated sodium channels in the postsynaptic membrane, thereby increasing the effective coupling of local EPPs and muscle fiber action potentials [2].

Q. Zhou, J. Chen, *Ocular Myasthenia Gravis*, Experts' Perspectives on Medical Advances,
https://doi.org/10.1007/978-981-96-1245-1_2

The pathophysiological mechanism of MG is related to the destruction of the normal structure and function of NMJ. The structure of the postsynaptic membrane of a healthy NMJ is highly ordered and tightly folded, with AChR densely distributed at the top of these folds, and voltage-gated sodium channels concentrated in the grooves. The normal aggregation of AChR depends on various structural proteins, such as low-density lipoprotein receptor-related protein 4 (LRP4) and muscle-specific tyrosine kinase receptor (MuSK), etc. [2]. The NMJ tissue structure is crucial for ensuring the precise coupling of EPPs and AP generation. Under conditions of continuous nerve activity, the amount of ACh released from the presynaptic membrane of a healthy NMJ gradually decreases, a normal physiological phenomenon known as "synaptic fatigue." Due to the safety factor of a healthy NMJ, EPPs can still maintain a large enough amplitude to trigger AP. However, in OMG patients, NMJ dysfunction leads to a significant reduction or complete loss of the safety factor, thereby greatly reducing the amplitude of mEPPs and EPPs, causing EPPs to fall below the threshold and fail to trigger AP to achieve muscle fiber excitation [4]. In addition to the reduction of EPPs, the decrease in the level of voltage-gated sodium channels in the postsynaptic membrane will also cause the threshold for inducing AP in MG to increase [5]. This inefficient neuromuscular transmission is manifested as a weakened response of compound motor action potentials (CMAPs) during repetitive nerve electrical stimulation [6], as well as abnormal jitter or blockage in single fiber electromyography [4, 7]. Clinically, this muscle response weakening accompanied by continuous nerve activity manifests as muscle weakness and is accompanied by characteristic fatigue [8].

2.2 Production of OMG Autoantibodies

It is crucial to delve into the source of autoantibodies, as the cells that produce these antibodies are potential therapeutic targets. Antibodies are mainly produced by specific antigen-activated B cell subgroups, including short-lived plasmablasts and long-lived plasma cells. The activation of B cells often requires the assistance of T cells; therefore, OMG is classified as a B cell-mediated T cell-dependent autoimmune disease. However, we still face many challenges and deficiencies in understanding the cellular immunology of OMG. Each B cell undergoes gene recombination of immunoglobulin gene variability (V), diversity (D), and joining (J) gene segments in the early stage of B cell development in the bone marrow during its development process, randomly producing one type of B cell receptor (BCR)/antibody, thereby forming up to 10^{11} unique B cell clones [7]. These clones can produce potentially harmful clones that express autoantibodies, thereby recognizing self-antigens and possibly triggering autoimmune responses [7]. Therefore, in the process of B cell maturation, there are two key "tolerance checkpoints," corresponding to central tolerance and peripheral tolerance. Central tolerance mainly occurs in the bone marrow and thymus, where the bone marrow and thymus are responsible for negative selection of self-antigens. This selection process, through mechanisms such as clonal deletion, induced incompetence, or receptor editing, aims to eliminate those B cells with potential polyreactive autoreactivity, thereby ensuring the self-tolerance and stability of the immune system. In addition, peripheral tolerance mainly occurs in peripheral immune organs such as the spleen, further precisely regulating the reactivity and specificity of B cells. These tolerance mechanisms together maintain the balance of the immune system, prevent excessive attack on self-tissues and also ensure that the immune system can effectively respond to the threat of foreign antigens [7, 9]. Studies have performed deep sequencing on the BCR library of AChR-Ab positive, MuSK-Ab positive MG, and healthy subjects, and found that there are a large number of abnormal immature cells and memory B cells in the peripheral blood of MG patients, suggesting that abnormal B cell receptor editing may promote the formation of autoreactive B cells [10]. In addition, further studies have shown that the frequency of polyreactive and autoreactive B cells in AChR-Ab and MuSK-Ab positive MG patients is higher than that in healthy controls, suggesting that there is a negative selection defect in MG patients, leading to autoreactive B cells escaping the control of tolerance checkpoints [11]. Based on this observation, the risk of MG patients suffering from other autoimmune diseases (i.e., polyautoimmunity) is significantly increased, with thyroid diseases being the most common [12]. These findings not only enrich our understanding of the pathogenesis of OMG, but also provide new ideas for future treatment strategies.

The activation of B cells depends on the assistance of T cells that can recognize the same antigen, and the negative selection process of autoreactive T cells is considered to be more stringent. T cells undergo negative selection against self-antigens in the thymus, especially in the medullary region of the thymus. In this process, autoimmune regulators (AIRE) play a key role in maintaining central tolerance [13, 14]. These autoimmune regulators can induce ectopic expression of self-reactive antigens in thymic stromal cells (such as medullary thymic epithelial cells (mTEC)). Subsequently, these self-reactive antigens are directly presented to developing T cells by mTEC, or indirectly presented through antigen-presenting cells [15, 16]. If developing T cells bind strongly to these self-reactive antigens, they are cleared from the immune cell pool through mechanisms such as clonal deletion, induced incompetence, or transformation into regulatory T cells (Tregs) with immunoregulatory and anti-inflammatory functions. Studies have reported that thymic abnormalities such as follicular hyperplasia or thymoma can impair central tolerance mechanisms, thereby facilitating AChR-specific helper T cells (Th) evade tolerance control [17]. In the pathogenesis of MG, these escaped AChR-specific Th cells activate AChR-specific B cells to produce AChR-Ab [18-20]. Changes in thymus function lead to an increase in the release of autoreactive CD4+T cells and CD8+T cells, leading to an imbalance in T cell subgroups [19, 21, 22]. In the ectopic germinal centers in the thymus, an increase in the number of Th cells is observed, which play a key role in the selection and survival of B cells [23, 24]. In addition, Th17 cells play an important role in autoimmune inflammation and tissue damage, and there is evidence that they may also play an important pathogenic role in the pathogenesis of MG [25-28]. In MG patients, an increase in the number of Th1/Th17 cells is observed, leading to a change in cytokine balance, manifested as an increase in Th1/Th17 cytokine levels and a decrease in IL-10 levels [28, 29]. On the other hand, Tregs, as key participants in maintaining peripheral self-tolerance, are impaired in MG and cannot effectively inhibit the ex vivo activation of T cells [30]. Further research shows that the number of Tregs in MG patients is reduced [31-33], further exacerbating the imbalance of immune tolerance.

In summary, the antibody production process in OMG patients involves abnormal regulation of B cells, T cell subgroups, and changes in cytokine balance, providing an important theoretical basis for a deeper understanding of the pathogenesis of this disease and the development of potential treatment strategies.

2.3 Role of Antibodies in OMG

In OMG, several pathogenic autoantibodies against different components of the NMJ have been found. Among them, the acetylcholine receptor antibody (AChR-Ab) against AChR is the most common, which can cause complement-mediated postsynaptic membrane destruction [34]. In addition, AChR-Ab not only blocks the action of ACh but also causes AChR cross-linking, thereby accelerating receptor degradation. Another pathogenic antibody is the muscle-specific tyrosine kinase receptor antibody (MuSK-Ab), which is an IgG4 subtype antibody that does not activate the complement. Given the key role of MuSK in maintaining presynaptic and postsynaptic structure and function, MuSK-Ab interferes with normal MuSK activity, leading to a decrease in ACh release and inhibition of normal AChR aggregation [35]. Another antibody is the low-density lipoprotein receptor-related protein 4 antibody (LRP4-Ab), further impairs NMJ function by interfering with MuSK activation and signal transduction, as well as complement activation and postsynaptic membrane destruction [36]. In this section, we will delve into the immunopathological mechanisms of the most common antibodies associated with OMG.

2.3.1 Pathogenic Mechanism of Acetylcholine Receptor Antibody (AChR-Ab)

The muscle AChR of NMJ is the main target of antibody attack in MG patients. More than 60 years ago, Del Castillo and Katz first discovered that AChR is located at NMJ [37]. Ultrastructural studies of Torpedo californica electric organ membrane preparations revealed the hexagonal structural features of AChR, and it was speculated that it was a ring structure composed of six receptor subunits [38]. However, subsequent research confirmed that AChR is actually a pentamer composed of five receptor subunits [39]. With further research, AChR has undergone a large amount of purification and biochemical characterization work [40]. By the 1980s, AChR genes were successively cloned, first from Torpedo, and then the corresponding genes were successfully cloned in rodents and humans [41].

Muscle AChR is a transmembrane pentameric structure, containing two developmental regulatory subtypes, namely embryonic/fetal AChR and adult AChR. The embryonic/fetal AChR glycoprotein is composed of five subunits, namely 2 α, 1 β, 1 γ, and 1 δ subunit. In adult AChR, the γ subunit is replaced by the ε subunit, forming the α2βεδ combination [42]. Each subunit contains a highly structured extracellular domain (ECD), four transmembrane domains, and an intracellular domain. AChR-Ab can target the ECD of different subunits of AChR, thus showing significant heterogeneity [20, 42]. Studies have shown that about half of AChR-Ab binds to the α subunit, especially the main immunogenic region on the ECD of the α subunit, the core of which is located between the amino acid fragments 67–76, and other amino acid fragments can also bind to the α subunit [42]. Further research has also found that AChR-Ab against the α subunit has stronger pathogenicity than antibodies against other subunits [43].

Based on the thymocyte-related immunoglobulin sequence, researchers successfully cloned the first batch of recombinant AChR-specific autoantibodies [44]. In addition, several AChR-specific human monoclonal antibodies were produced by various methods [45]. These recombinant human monoclonal antibodies simulate the characteristics of serum AChR-Ab, compete with the AChR region recognized by autoantibodies in the serum [44], and their pathogenic characteristics have been proven by passive transfer MG experiments [45].

These monoclonal antibodies, together with studies of AChR-Ab derived from human serum, have revealed three main pathogenic mechanisms of AChR-Ab. These mechanisms mainly achieve their effects by reducing the number or function of muscle AChR [46], specifically including: (1) Complement activation: AChR-Ab mainly belongs to IgG1 and IgG3 subclasses, which can effectively activate the complement system, leading to the formation of the membrane attack complex (MAC), which in turn destroys the postsynaptic folds of NMJ, causing focal lysis, and ultimately leading to the destruction of AChR and its related proteins (i.e., rapsyn and voltage-gated sodium channels) at the endplate [47]. The successful application of complement inhibitors (such as eculizumab) in the treatment of refractory MG patients further confirms the key role of complement in AChR MG pathology [48]. (2) Antigen modulation: Autoantibodies can mediate the cross-linking of adjacent AChRs, thereby accelerating their internalization and degradation. The bivalent structure of the antibody allows it to bind to two AChR molecules through two antigen-binding sites, leading to receptor cross-linking and accelerated removal from the cell surface, thereby reducing the number of AChRs at the NMJ [49]. (3) Blocking the binding of acetylcholine to AChR: AChR-Ab can occupy the binding site on the surface of AChR or the area close to the binding site, thereby preventing the normal binding of acetylcholine to the receptor, inhibiting NMJ site acetylcholine-dependent signal transmission.

Patients positive for AChR-Ab often do not express only a single monoclonal antibody group. Due to the heterogeneity of the AChR-Ab response, these antibodies can be divided into three types: binding antibodies, blocking antibodies, and modulating antibodies [50]. Studies have shown that the detection of AChR binding antibodies has extremely high sensitivity [51]. In 4740 serum samples of AChR-Ab positive MG, 88% of the samples detected binding antibodies, 70% detected modulating antibodies, and 65% detected blocking antibodies [51]. It is worth noting that early-onset MG (before 50 years old), GMG, and thymoma MG patients often present high levels of AChR binding antibodies [52]. In addition, there is also a correlation between thymoma and high levels of AChR modulating antibodies [53]. Kang et al. pointed out that when only blocking antibodies or binding antibodies are detected, patients often present as OMG and mild GMG. Both binding antibodies and blocking antibodies are related to the severity of the disease in MG patients [50]. Especially in severe GMG or thymoma patients, they often have high titers of both AChR binding antibodies and blocking antibodies, usually indicating a poor prognosis [50]. However, some studies have shown that patients with severe myasthenia gravis have lower antibody titers, while some patients in remission or with only ocular manifestations have higher antibody titers [54]. These seemingly contradictory results actually reflect the heterogeneity of AChR-Ab in terms of specificity, affinity, and isotype. In addition, different patients may have different subtypes of AChR-Ab, which also differ in their pathogenicity. Nevertheless, the detection of binding-type AChR-Ab is generally considered the most useful auxiliary examination for diagnosing MG, while the determination of regulatory antibodies and blocking antibodies is relatively small in diagnostic sensitivity.

In most studies, there was no consistent correlation between the concentrations of AChR-Ab in different individuals and the severity of the disease [54]. However, studies have shown that there is a correlation between AChR epitope variability and disease severity [43]; therefore, identifying the binding regions and subclasses of antibodies may help enhance this correlation. Compared to the detection of total antibody concentration, the concentration of antibodies against the main immunogenic region has a stronger correlation with disease severity [54]. In addition, AChR-Ab titer can also serve as a risk assessment indicator for transient neonatal MG (TNMG). Specifically, when the maternal titer exceeds 100 nM, the risk of TNMG increases; when the titer is below 10 nM, the risk is relatively low [55]. In a cohort study involving 75 MG patients, continuous monitoring of AChR-Ab found that, after treatment with prednisone or immunosuppressants and thymectomy, most patients' symptoms improved with the decrease of AChR-Ab titer [56]. On the contrary, this correlation is weaker in the absence of immunosuppressive treatment [57]. Therefore, testing serial samples from the same patient is important for monitoring disease progression and guiding disease management.

The AChR-Ab titer in OMG patients is usually lower than in GMG patients [58]. More importantly, there is a significant correlation between higher AChR-Ab titer and the risk of GMG conversion [58]. The study by Peeler et al. showed that the AChR antibody titer (measured by RIPA method) was significantly higher in OMG patients who converted to GMG than in those who did not, with average concentrations of 12.7 nmol/L and 4.2 nmol/L, respectively [58]. Subsequently, Feng et al. measured the AChR-Ab titer in 19 OMG patients in the Chinese population and found through statistical analysis that when the AChR-Ab titer (measured by ELISA method) reached or exceeded 6.13 nmol/L, it could serve as a predictive indicator for GMG conversion [59]. Recently, a study by Supawongwattana et al. measured the AChR-Ab titer in 118 Thai OMG patients and found that when the AChR-Ab titer reached or exceeded 8.11 nmol/L, the risk of OMG patients converting to GMG significantly increased, so these patients need to be closely monitored and reminded of the possible early symptoms of life-threatening GMG [60]. In addition, the study also pointed out that for AChR-Ab positive OMG patients, especially when the AChR-Ab titer is for patients with ≥2.81 nmol/L and ≥15.12 nmol/L, it is recommended to conduct serum thyroid autoantibody testing and chest CT for thymoma screening. In summary, these research results further enhance the value of AChR-Ab detection in clinical practice, reminding us that when treating AChR-Ab positive OMG patients, we should fully consider their AChR antibody titer levels to improve necessary related examinations and develop better treatment plans.

The sensitivity of AChR-Ab to systemic MG in adults is 85–90%, while in OMG cases, its sensitivity is relatively lower, about 50%–70%. In MG cases that occur in childhood, its sensitivity is further reduced, only about 50%. However, in thymoma-related OMG patients, the sensitivity of AChR-Ab significantly increases, close to 100%. Regarding specificity, AChR-Ab shows extremely high specificity for MG, ranging between 95% and 100%. This high specificity stems from the negative results of AChR-Ab in healthy individuals and its rare occurrence in other autoimmune or neuromuscular diseases.

Serological testing of AChR-Ab is usually the first step in diagnosing OMG. Currently, the Radioimmunoprecipitation Assay (RIPA) is the most widely used method for AChR-Ab detection [61]. RIPA has very high specificity (about 99%) and sensitivity (about 85% in GMG, about 50% in OMG) and is considered the gold standard for detecting AChR-Ab [62]. As a quantitative method, RIPA can effectively monitor changes in antibody concentrations in individual patients by measuring antibody levels. However, the application of RIPA is limited because it uses radioactive reagents. Therefore, the radiation hazards associated with it limit its use in personnel without special training and laboratories without radiation permits. With the advancement of technology, non-radioactive detection methods have emerged and been commercialized. Among them, the Enzyme-Linked Immunosorbent Assay (ELISA), due to its performance close to RIPA, has become the preferred option for laboratories that cannot perform radioactive detection. Another non-radioactive alternative to RIPA is the Fluorescent Immunoprecipitation Method (FIPA), which uses fluorescently labeled target antigens. Although FIPA has been proven to have relatively good overall sensitivity and specificity, it is still slightly inferior to RIPA. Although FIPA avoids the hazards of radioactivity, its operation requires specific equipment and professional knowledge, so its application in routine diagnosis is limited [63]. In the past decade, Cell-Based Assays (CBA) have also been introduced into MG diagnosis. CBA uses transiently or stably co-transfected cells, these plasmids encode the five subunits of nicotinic acetylcholine receptor (nAChR) and rapsyn. Through co-transfection, natural nAChR is overexpressed on the cell membrane, simulating the densely clustered nAChR on the neuromuscular junction (NMJ). Therefore, CBA surpasses RIPA and ELISA based on purified AChR molecules in detection sensitivity. CBA can not only provide semi-quantitative evaluation of autoantibody titers, but also perform quantitative analysis through flow cytometry. Studies have shown that the sensitivity of CBA is higher than RIPA, and its specificity is close to 100% [64]. It has been reported that 38.1%–66% of serum antibody negative MG patients found autoantibodies against clustered nAChR in CBA testing [64]. In addition, CBA detected AChR-Ab in 50% of AChR-Ab negative OMG patients [65]. CBA not only provides higher sensitivity for the diagnosis of OMG, but also avoids the radiation hazards associated with RIPA. Therefore, more and more patients who were previously considered to be serum antibody negative are now diagnosed through CBA. It is worth noting that studies have found that patients who are detected with AChR-Ab only through CBA often show milder symptoms and better treatment effects [64].

2.3.2 Pathogenesis of Muscle-Specific Tyrosine Kinase Receptor Antibody (MuSK-Ab)

In 2001, Werner Hoch et al. [66] first successfully detected MuSK-Ab in AChR-Ab negative MG serum. MuSK was initially identified as a novel

Trk-related tyrosine kinase receptor [67]. Subsequently, MuSK-Ab was isolated as a gene product and was significantly induced in the process of denervation of mouse muscles [68]. Although MuSK was initially thought to be expressed only in skeletal muscle, hence the name muscle-specific kinase, subsequent research has shown that MuSK is also distributed in other tissues and cells [69].

MuSK is a transmembrane protein that is closely related to the cytoskeletal structure of the postsynaptic membrane. It contains extracellular, transmembrane helical, and cytoplasmic domains, and has tyrosine kinase activity. Its extracellular domain characteristically includes three immunoglobulin-like regions and a cysteine-rich coiled-coil domain. Following the transmembrane region is a short juxtamembrane region, a tyrosine kinase domain, and a C-terminal sequence of eight amino acids. Huijbers et al. [70] and Koneczny et al. [71] revealed its potential pathogenic mechanism: MuSK-Ab binds to the N-terminus of the MuSK extracellular domain, thereby preventing the interaction of MuSK with LRP4, and inhibiting Agrin-induced AChR clustering.

Unlike AChR-Ab, MuSK-Ab mainly belongs to the IgG4 subclass and does not activate complement [72]. Complement activation is not necessary in the pathogenesis of MG, and both bivalent and monovalent antibodies may induce MG in vivo by inducing MuSK dysfunction [73, 74]. Further research found that purified IgG4 from MuSK-Ab positive MG patients can bind to mouse neuromuscular junctions in vitro and induce myasthenia gravis after injection into immunodeficient mice. These mice have reduced AChR density and fragmentation at the neuromuscular junction. Electrophysiological synaptic analysis further revealed that postsynaptic ACh sensitivity is severely reduced, and presynaptic ACh release is excessively inhibited during high-rate activity, both of which lead to fatigable muscle weakness [75]. The results indicate that MuSK-Ab has both presynaptic and postsynaptic effects on neuromuscular transmission, and these effects do not depend on complement activation [74].

Research shows that MuSK IgG blocks the binding of MuSK to the collagen tail (Collagen Q or ColQ) of the end-plate acetylcholinesterase, and the binding of ColQ to MuSK is crucial for promoting AChR aggregation [76]. This finding reveals at least in some patients that the main target of MuSK-Ab is ColQ, which may explain the experimental observation that acetylcholinesterase inhibitors (ACEIs) are ineffective in mouse models [73], and is also consistent with clinical observations that ACEIs have limited efficacy in many MuSK-Ab positive MG patients [77].

In the detection of MG patients, about 6% of patients detected the presence of MuSK-Ab [78]. In AChR-Ab negative GMG cases, the sensitivity of MuSK-Ab ranges between 5% and 70% [79, 80], and it is usually difficult to detect in OMG patients [81]. This ratio varies between different geographical regions, with Nordic countries having a relatively low positivity rate for MuSK-Ab, and the Mediterranean region having a higher positivity rate, which may be attributed to geographical and genetic differences. Notably, MuSK-Ab positive MG cases are relatively rare in the Japanese population, with an overall prevalence of 2%–3% [82]. In the past, the detection of MuSK-Ab in AChR-Ab positive patients was very rare [83, 84]. However, in the Chinese population, it has been reported that 4% of AChR-Ab negative MG patients and 2.3%–5.9% of AChR-Ab positive MG patients detected the presence of MuSK-Ab [85, 86, 87]. The specificity of MuSK-Ab is extremely high, usually between 94% and 100%, so false positive results are relatively few [88]. Compared with AChR-Ab, there is a significant correlation between the titer level of MuSK-Ab and the severity of the disease, both in individual cases and in the entire population [57, 89]. A possible explanation for this correlation is that most MuSK-Ab primarily targets the first IgG-like domain, which contrasts sharply with the heterogeneity of AChR-Ab. Patients positive for MuSK-Ab are more likely to have refractory MG and symptoms of respiratory weakness [90]. These patients often have an inadequate response to ACEIs treatment, and sometimes the condition may worsen after receiving bromide treatment. In addition, MuSK-Ab positive patients usually respond better to plasma exchange than to intravenous immunoglobulin [91].

Regarding the laboratory method for detecting MuSK-Ab, RIPA is an immunoprecipitation technique involving co-incubation with patient serum of the 125I-MuSK extracellular domain, and is currently considered the gold standard for MG antibody identification [92]. 80%–85% of MG patient serum AChR-Ab is positive, while only 5%–7% of MG patients are positive for MuSK-Ab [93]. To enhance the sensitivity of RIPA, a two-step alternative detection method has been developed: first, affinity chromatography is used to concentrate the potentially extremely low titer of MuSK-Ab from a large amount of serum; the second step is to use standard RIPA for detection [94]. It is worth noting that this method requires the use of serum diluted 50 times in volume to avoid the impact of increased nonspecific binding.

Although commercially available ELISA for detecting MuSK-Ab is available, it is not the first choice. As a non-radioactive alternative to RIPA, FIPA has shown great potential, and the sensitivity of these two detection methods has been proven to be equivalent [63]. Importantly, FIPA achieves simultaneous detection of AChR-Ab and MuSK-Ab by labeling each antigen with different fluorescent dyes, thereby reducing the cost and time of diagnosis.

To avoid radioactivity and increase sensitivity, researchers have developed a CBA method for detecting MuSK-Ab. CBA has shown high sensitivity and specificity in detecting autoantibodies in MuSK-Ab positive MG patients, which is mainly attributed to the antigen being expressed in a more natural conformation and easier to recognize [95, 96]. Using the CBA method, researchers even detected MuSK-Ab in the serum of patients with serum AChR-Ab negative, including Asians [63, 79, 85, 97]. An international study tested the serum of 633 serum negative MG (SNMG) patients from 13 European countries, and the results showed that the prevalence of MuSK-Ab was 5%–22% [81]. The CBA data in this study showed that MuSK-Ab positive MG is more common in OMG patients than previously thought. In a recent study in Korea, CBA's sensitivity in detecting MuSK-Ab exceeded that of traditional RIPA [98]. Other studies have also shown that when the CBA method is used to detect MuSK-Ab, the positive rate of MuSK-Ab in MG patients is higher than that of RIPA [85, 98, 99]. Studies have shown that neither patients with other neuromuscular diseases nor healthy people showed positive results for MuSK-Ab in CBA testing [98]. In addition, CBA can also detect MuSK-Ab positive cases that were previously considered to be MuSK-Ab negative or borderline cases based on RIPA. These results indicate that CBA has high sensitivity and specificity for detecting MuSK-Ab. Although the CBA method involves cell culture, DNA transfection, and fluorescence microscopy, these techniques can be implemented in most laboratories, and they are more stable and safer than radioactive compounds, so the CBA method is increasingly used in routine testing.

2.3.3 Pathogenic Mechanism of Low-Density Lipoprotein Receptor-Related Protein 4 Antibody (LPR4-Ab)

LRP4 has been widely recognized as the third autoimmune target in MG patients, playing a crucial role in synapse development and maintenance. LRP4 is a single-pass transmembrane protein with a large extracellular domain, which includes 8 low-density lipoprotein receptor class A repeat sequences, 2 EGF-like domains, and 4 β-propeller (β-propeller, BP) domains, each BP domain is combined with an EGF-like domain [100]. In biological processes, neural Agrin primarily binds with the first BP structural domain of LRP4, and subsequent LDLa repeats also contribute to this binding [101]. LRP4 acts as a muscle receptor for the Agrin protein, forming an LRP4-Agrin complex, which then binds and activates MuSK, thereby promoting the aggregation of AChR at the neuromuscular junction [100]. Notably, pathogenic LRP4 antibodies belong to the IgG1/IgG2 subclass, which have the ability to activate the complement cascade, block LRP4-

Agrin signal transduction, cause MuSK inactivation, and inhibit the aggregation of AChR at the neuromuscular junction [102].

Regarding the positive detection rate of LRP4-Ab in MG patients, there is a significant difference between different studies (2%–45%), which may be due to the use of different detection methods (such as ELISA, CBA or immunoprecipitation), antigen sources (animal or human), and the heterogeneity of the studied population (such as Japanese or Caucasians) [103-105]. A multinational study used CBA to analyze 635 patient samples that did not detect AChR-Ab or MuSK-Ab and found that 19% of the patients had LRP4-Ab, which is equivalent to 2% of all MG patients, and there are significant regional differences between different countries, from 7% in Norway and Turkey to 33% in Poland [106]. Studies on the Chinese population show that the positive rate of LRP4-Ab is lower than in Western countries, only found in 0.8%–1.7% of MG patients and 1%–2.9% of seronegative (i.e., both AChR-Ab and MuSK-Ab are negative) MG patients and is mainly related to OMG [107, 108]. However, it is worth noting that LRP4-Ab also exists in about 8% of AChR-Ab positive patients, 15%–20% of MuSK positive patients, and 3.6% of patients with other neurological diseases [81, 106, 109]. In addition, the prevalence of LRP4-Ab in patients with amyotrophic lateral sclerosis has been reported, ranging from 10% to 23% [98]. Therefore, simply detecting LRP4-Ab in the patient's blood may not be sufficient to establish a diagnosis of OMG, and a comprehensive analysis must be combined with the patient's clinical manifestations. More in-depth research is still needed to determine the specificity and clinical utility of LRP4-Ab in the diagnosis of OMG [110, 111].

Given the important role of LRP4-Ab in the pathogenesis of MG, it is recommended to detect serum LRP4-Ab in seronegative patients through CBA (using HEK293 cells transfected with LRP4 recombinant protein) or ELISA. However, in CBA, the expression of LRP4 transmembrane protein has always faced challenges [62]. Studies have shown that when co-expressed with Mesoderm development candidate 2 (Mesdc2), the transport efficiency of LRP4 to the cell surface is significantly improved [1, 112]. In addition, quantitative detection of LRP4-Ab has also been optimized through flow cytometry.

2.4 Role of Immune Cells in OMG

OMG is a subtype of MG, and the mechanism of action of immune cells in OMG is consistent with MG [98]. It is currently believed that when the body's immune tolerance mechanism is damaged, antigen-presenting cells (APC) will actively uptake self-antigens such as AChR. These antigens are then finely processed within the APC, combined with the major histocompatibility complex, forming an antigen-major histocompatibility complex compound. This compound is then specifically recognized by $CD4^+$ T cell receptors (TCR), triggering a series of complex and orderly immune responses. In this process, the expression levels of a series of cytokines, such as IL-4 and IL-6, are significantly upregulated. These cytokines play a crucial role in regulating B cells to differentiate into plasma cells and memory cells, thereby promoting the production of AChR-Ab. In the end-plate region of NMJ, AChR-Ab specifically binds to AChR, and then, with the participation of the complement, accelerates the degradation process of AChR. Due to the massive destruction of AChR, the endplate cannot generate enough end-plate potential, leading to impaired synaptic transmission, ultimately causing symptoms of myasthenia gravis. In addition, activated T cells can also secrete pro-inflammatory cytokines, such as IFN-γ and IL-17. These cytokines further promote antibody production by regulating the balance between regulatory T cells (Treg) and Th17 cells [113].

The synthesis of high-affinity pathogenic AChR-Ab requires the participation of $CD4^+$ T helper cells and their secreted cytokines, which play a crucial role in the development and regulation of autoimmune responses [114]. Previous studies believed that the pathogenesis of MG is related to T helper cells (Th), especially the imbalance of Th1 and Th2 cell expression, leading to the production of a large number of autoantibodies. With the continuous deepening of theoretical research, the imbalance theory of Th1/Th2 cells cannot objectively and accurately explain the pathogenesis of MG [115]. Recent studies have found that initial $CD4^+$ T cells differentiate into Tregs under the induction of transforming growth factor β1 (TGF-β1), participating in immune regulation; or differentiate into T helper cells 17 (Th17) under the joint induction of interleukin 6 (IL-6) and TGF-β, participating in inflammatory responses and autoimmune diseases [116, 117]. With the deepening of MG research, Treg cells and Th17 cells are also involved in the occurrence and development of MG. The imbalance of Th17/Treg cell expression is a key factor in the pathogenesis of MG [98].

As a newly discovered functional $CD4^+$ T cell subgroup, Th17 cells are usually regarded as inflammatory Th cell subgroups. Th17 cells can specifically express IL-17 to participate in immune tolerance, maintain tissue or organ homeostasis, and receive widespread attention in autoimmune diseases. In MG research, $CD4^+$ Research on T cell subgroups has shown that, compared with the healthy control group, the concentration of IL-17 is increased in both AChR-Ab positive and negative MG patients, and the number of Th17 cells also shows an increasing trend. This finding suggests that Th17 cells play an important role in the pathogenesis of MG [98]. Further research has found that there is a significant positive correlation between the number of Th17 cells in the peripheral blood of MG patients and the concentration of AChR-Ab, and it is closely related to the severity of the disease and the score of the myasthenia gravis quantitative table [98]. In experimental autoimmune myasthenia gravis (EAMG), researchers also observed a significant increase in the expression of IL-17 and the proportion of Th17 cells, further emphasizing the importance of IL-17 in the pathogenesis of EAMG [118]. In recent years, research has also revealed the role of Th17 cells in regulating the balance of Th1/Th2 cell factors. Under the stimulation of Th17 cells, B cells can quickly synthesize and secrete immunoglobulins, and when the amount of immunoglobulins reaches a certain level, it will accelerate the onset of MG [119]. In addition, research on thymic hyperplasia in MG patients has found that the activation of the IL-23/Th17 pathway not only leads to inflammation, but also maintains the activity of the thymic germinal center [120]. In summary, Th17 cells play a crucial role in the pathogenesis of MG.

Treg cells are a subgroup of T cells that inhibit the body's immune response and are key cells in suppressing autoimmune responses. Treg cells mainly exert their immunosuppressive and immune-stabilizing characteristics by inhibiting the activation and proliferation of autoreactive T cells present in the normal body [121]. Fattorossi et al. [122] found that the number of circulating Treg cells in untreated MG patients is lower than that in healthy subjects, and in MG patients treated with prednisone and azathioprine, the number of Treg cells is normal or increased. This suggests that the lack of Treg cells is conducive to the development of MG, and its normalization is an important clinical observation indicator for immunosuppressive treatment. In addition, Luther et al. [83] reported that compared with untreated MG patients, the in vitro immunosuppressive function of Treg in MG patients treated with prednisolone is enhanced, indicating that prednisolone may enhance the function of Treg, which is consistent with the research results of Fattorossi et al. [122]. In EAMG, Aricha et al. [123] also observed that the number of circulating Treg cells is lower than that in the healthy control group, which further indicates that Treg cells play a key role in controlling myasthenia gravis. The key transcription factor and specific marker of Treg cells, FOXP3, regulates the activity of Treg by regulating multiple genes. The immunosuppressive effect of Treg cells depends on immunoregulatory cytokines such as IL-10 [124]. The expression levels of FOXP3 and IL-10 in the serum of MG patients are significantly reduced, suggesting that there may be functional defects in the Treg cell subgroup [124]. After single tacrolimus treatment in MG patients, the detection of peripheral blood mononuclear cells (PBMC) revealed an increase in the expression of Treg cells, and the originally low expression level of IL-10 was also restored [115]. In addition, the expression of FOXP3 is regulated to some extent by signals induced by the IL-2 transduction pathway and the phosphorylation of transcription activation protein 5. Existing research reports that the levels of IL-2 in the thymus and serum of MG patients have increased [125]. These findings provide a new perspective for us to understand the role of Treg cells in the pathogenesis of MG and also provide a theoretical basis for potential treatment strategies.

When discussing the balance regulation between Th17 cells and Treg cells, the role of IL-6 is particularly important [84]. When the body faces the challenge of infection or inflammation, the expression of IL-6 may excessively rise or the regulation mechanism may become abnormal. In this process, other key pro-inflammatory factors, such as IL-1β, IL-21, IL-23, and TNF-α, will also participate in the process of cell differentiation and jointly promote the expression of IL-6. These pro-inflammatory factors inhibit the generation of Treg cells and jointly act on the differentiation process of Th17 cells with TGF-β, thereby inducing the body's inflammatory response [86]. Souroujon MC and others [87] further confirmed the regulatory role of IL-6 in the imbalance of Th17/Treg cells through the study of the EAMG model, and the injection of IL-6 antibodies can alleviate and improve myasthenia gravis symptoms. In addition, the serum of AChR-Ab positive MG patients was tested, and the results showed that the level of IL-6 in these patients was significantly higher than that of normal people, further supporting the important role of IL-6 in regulating the imbalance of Th17/Treg cells, and suggesting its potential therapeutic value as a key target for regulating MG autoimmune responses [126, 127].

Myeloid-derived suppressor cells (MDSCs) are a heterogeneous group of immature myeloid cells that play a key role in the pathogenesis of cancer and various chronic inflammatory diseases [128]. These cells have the ability to suppress T cell responses, thereby promoting the progression and metastasis of tumors, and are therefore considered potential therapeutic targets for cancer [129]. Regarding the inhibitory effect of MDSCs in EAMG, in-depth studies have been conducted in mouse models [130]. Transplantation of MDSCs significantly improved the symptoms of myasthenia gravis in experimental mice, and the levels of AChR-Ab IgG in the serum and terminal complement deposition both decreased. Further analysis showed that the levels of IFN-γ and IL-17 produced by mouse spleen cells treated with MDSCs in vitro were reduced, indicating that MDSCs can effectively inhibit Th1 and Th17 immune responses. In addition, MDSCs can directly inhibit pre-activated B cells in vitro an in vivo. In summary, MDSCs inhibit the development of EAMG by suppressing autoreactive T cells and B cells [130]. These findings not only deepen our understanding of the mechanism of action of MDSCs in EAMG, but also provide important clues for the development of new therapeutic targets in the future.

B regulatory cells (Bregs), a heterogeneous population of immunosuppressive B cells, have been extensively studied in humans and mice, primarily suppressing inflammatory responses through the synthesis of IL-10. Multiple studies have shown that compared to healthy controls, untreated AChR-Ab positive MG patients show a decrease in the number and function of circulating Bregs [95, 131]. Thymectomy can restore the proportion of circulating Bregs, but steroid treatment does not achieve this effect [149. Further research focuses on a specific subset of Bregs—IL-10 producing B cells (B10 cells) [130]. For patients treated with rituximab, the therapeutic effect is significantly related to the proliferation rate of B10 cells. In patients who respond well to rituximab treatment, their B10 cells show a rapid re-proliferation ability, while in patients who do not respond well to rituximab, B10 cell re-proliferation is delayed [131]. In addition, Guptill et al. [95] reported that compared to healthy controls, the number of B10 cells in MuSK-Ab positive MG patients is significantly reduced. Therefore, in AChR-Ab positive and MuSK-Ab positive MG, the reduction in the number of Bregs is closely related to the immunopathogenic role.

In summary, although these studies provide us with some new insights into the pathogenesis of OMG, the specific functions and interaction mechanisms of these cells in OMG still need to be further explored. Therefore, future research should focus on comprehensively analyzing the roles of various regulatory cells in OMG, in order to provide new strategies and methods for disease treatment.

2.5 Role of Complement in OMG

AChR-Ab binds to AChR at the NMJ, leading to the internalization of AChR and activation of the complement system [96, 132]. This activation process involves the classical and alternative pathways, jointly mediating the formation of MAC. The direct effect of MAC is to damage the postsynaptic membrane of the NMJ, leading to a reduction in the area of secondary folds of the postsynaptic membrane, and thus reducing the number of AChR and voltage-gated sodium channels on the endplate [96]. This damage interferes with the signal transmission between nerves and muscles, ultimately leading to symptoms of muscle weakness [96]. Complement components (such as C3 and C9) are deposited at the NMJ of MG patients, these deposits are direct evidence of complement activation and MAC formation [99]. Studies have found that the levels of C3 and/or C4 in the serum of MG patients are significantly reduced, especially in cases with high levels of AChR-Ab, indicating that AChR-Ab may overconsume factors of the classical and common complement pathways [133]. Tüzün et al. [96] found that in some patients with myasthenia gravis where serological tests show negative AChR-Ab or normal electromyography, there are deposits of IgG, complement C3 and C9 at the neuromuscular junction. In addition, Yang et al. [134] the involvement of the complement system in the pathogenesis of OMG was also found to be confirmed in a model of experimental autoimmune myasthenia gravis in extraocular muscles. Wu et al. [135, 136] further found that HLA-DQ8 transgenic mice immunized with human-derived AChRγ subunit showed susceptibility to OMG, and HLA-DR3 transgenic mice immunized with human-derived AChRε subunit were also susceptible to OMG. This difference in susceptibility to OMG may be closely related to the deposition of IgG, C3, and membrane attack complex at the neuromuscular junction of the extraocular muscle [96].

Due to its unique physiological characteristics and high metabolic demand, the extraocular muscle is more susceptible to MG than other muscles. More importantly, the extraocular muscle seems to have a higher sensitivity to complement-mediated damage [137]. This phenomenon may be related to the reduced expression of complement-related regulatory factors in the extraocular muscle. For example, the expression level of CD55 (also known as decay accelerating factor, DAF) in the extraocular muscle is lower than that in skeletal muscle, while the expression level of CD59 is relatively high [137]. In addition, the secondary fold area of the postsynaptic membrane of the NMJ in the extraocular muscle is smaller than that in other skeletal muscles, making the involvement of the complement more likely to cause extraocular muscle weakness [137]. Genomic analysis and continuous analysis of gene expression further revealed differences in the expression of complement regulatory factor genes in the classical and alternative pathways between the extraocular muscle and other skeletal muscles [137].

Clinical studies by Howard et al. [138] showed that Eculizumab can inhibit the splitting of complement C5, thereby effectively relieving the myasthenic symptoms of AChR-Ab positive MG patients. Complement activation is closely related to the worsening of MG, and changes in the levels of complement activation products (such as C3 breakdown product C3c) can serve as indicators of disease activity [138, 139]. These studies emphasize the potential of anti-complement therapy in MG, especially monoclonal antibodies against C5 (such as Eculizumab, Ravulizumab, and Zilucoplan), which can effectively inhibit the formation of MAC and show positive clinical effects in the treatment of MG [113].

2.6 Role of Thymus in OMG

AChR-Ab is mainly produced in the thymus, playing a crucial role in the pathogenesis of OMG. Normally, the thymus of an adult individual undergoes a degenerative process, however, about 70% of MG patients show pathological features of thymic follicular hyperplasia, and about 15% of patients have thymoma [140]. There is currently no clear description of the prevalence of thymic lesions in OMG patients.

The thymus is the main lymphoid organ for the development and maturation of T cells. As a key lymphoid organ for the development and maturation of T cells, the thymus contains a rich variety of cell types. Among them, thymic epithelial cells (TECs) are the most abundant cell population, further subdivided into cortical TECs (cTECs) and medullary TECs (mTECs) based on their location in the thymic cortex or medulla. cTECs play a decisive role in the positive selection process of T cells, while mTECs are responsible for inducing the negative selection of highly self-reactive T cells, which is crucial for establishing central self-tolerance [141]. The mixed expression of various self-antigens in the thymus is crucial for the negative selection of self-reactive T cells and the establishment of central tolerance [142]. In addition, self-reactive T cells also play a key pathogenic role in the pathogenesis of MG. Thymic epithelial cells can directly or through antigen-presenting cells present self-antigens to developing T cells. If developing T cells bind strongly to these antigens, self-reactive T cells are cleared through clonal deletion, induced incompetence, or conversion to Tregs with immunoregulatory and anti-inflammatory functions. It is worth noting that AChR and other muscle proteins, such as RYR and Titin, are expressed by thymic myoid cells and thymic epithelial cells [143]. Autoimmune regulatory factors play a key role in the autoimmune process of T cells, on the one hand, regulating the expression of peripheral tissue-restricted antigens of medullary TECs, thereby inducing the negative selection of self-reactive T cells; on the other hand, participating in the positive selection process of Tregs.

Thymic abnormalities in OMG patients, such as thymic follicular hyperplasia or thymoma, often lead to defects in central tolerance mechanisms and the escape of AChR-specific T cells [17]. These abnormalities include: (1) defects in the expression of autoimmune regulatory factors in mTECs [144, 145]; (2) estrogen down-regulates the transcription of autoimmune regulatory factors, which may explain the predominance of female patients [14, 146]; (3) absence of thymic medulla, and thymoma cells lack the ability for negative selection [147]; (4) proliferative or tumorous cTECs presenting self-antigens [148] or down-regulation of major histocompatibility complex (MHC) II expression [17]; (5) abnormal expression of pro-inflammatory cytokines. These mechanisms together lead to the dysfunction of T cell negative selection, thereby promoting the release of self-reactive CD4+T cells and CD8+T cells [149]. In addition, the imbalance of T cell subsets and cytokine dysregulation promote the activation of germinal center B cells, thereby activating AChR-specific B cells to produce autoantibodies [20].

There is a close association between OMG and thymic hyperplasia and thymoma. Thymic hyperplasia is a term for follicular hyperplasia in the thymus [150, 151], its main feature is the formation of ectopic germinal centers [152]. The attack of antibodies and complement on thymic myoid cells may lead to the formation of antigen-antibody complexes, which in turn stimulate antigen-presenting cells and induce the formation of ectopic germinal centers in the thymus [153]. Ectopic germinal centers in the MG thymus contribute to the differentiation of B cells into autoreactive memory B cells and plasma cells [154]. Studies have shown that B cells in the hyperplastic thymus of MG patients show an increase in memory B cells and potential autoreactive B cells [153]. In addition, compared with B cells in the thymus of the healthy control group, B cells in the MG thymus show a higher activation state [155]. Ectopic germinal centers in the thymus contain AChR-specific long-lived plasma cells that can produce high levels of AChR-Ab [156-158]. Thymoma is a rare tumor that originates from thymic epithelial cells and is bordered by T cells [159]. Because thymomas originate from cortical epithelial cells and lack antigen-presenting cells in the functional medulla involved in negative selection [159]; therefore, thymomas can produce autoreactive T cells, trigger autoimmune responses, reduce tolerance to AChR, and initiate the occurrence of AChR-Ab positive MG mediated by thymomas [160].

Thymectomy, as a treatment for MG, has shown significant therapeutic effects in the patient population related to thymoma-associated GMG, and can also effectively treat GMG cases with thymic hyperplasia [160]. Li et al. [161] further pointed out that early thymectomy for patients with thymoma or thymic hyperplasia can help reduce or even prevent the transformation of OMG to GMG. Shrager [162] proposed an exploratory view that for those refractory OMG patients without thymoma, thymectomy can also be used as a trial treatment. The British Myasthenia Gravis Guidelines made specific recommendations for certain patient groups, believing that OMG patients under 45 years old and AChR-Ab positive may increase the possibility of disease remission, reduce the risk of disease developing into systemic, and reduce dependence on corticosteroids after thymectomy [163]. However, although thymectomy has achieved long-term remission in some patients, about half (40%–50%) of AChR-Ab positive MG patients have achieved long-term remission after thymectomy and followed up for up to 20 years; however, some patients have not achieved complete remission [164, 165]. In MG patients who have undergone thymectomy, the titer of AChR-Ab generally shows a downward trend; however, the AChR-Ab level of some patients is still within the detectable range [120]. If surgery can completely remove all thymic tissue infiltrated by immunity, and the disease and autoantibodies persist, it strongly suggests that in addition to the thymus, there are B cells in other parts that can continuously produce autoantibodies. Research results show that B cells producing AChR-Ab can be found in the blood circulation and lymph nodes [166, 167]. The number of AChR-specific B cells in the blood circulation is usually positively correlated with thymic hyperplasia and high serum autoantibody titer [166]. In addition, there are B cells producing AChR-Ab in the bone marrow [168]. Long-lived plasma cells are plasma cells selected from the B cell pool with the highest affinity receptors, which can upregulate the expression of recombinant chemokine C-X-C-Motif Receptor 4(CXCR4), and migrate to the niche (usually in the bone marrow) to continue producing antibodies. Most serum immunoglobulins are produced by long-lived plasma cells and form serological memory. Therefore, plasma cells in the bone marrow that produce AChR-Ab may be an important factor for the continuous increase in antibody titer after thymectomy [169]. Although thymectomy can effectively eliminate the self-reactive B cells and their supporting cells in the thymus that have produced pathogenic AChR-Ab, the pathogenic B cells that have migrated from the thymus to peripheral immune organs (such as lymph nodes and bone marrow) may continue to stimulate disease activity [170]. Therefore, in the treatment and management of MG patients, in addition to thymectomy, the removal of pathogenic B cells in peripheral immune organs should also be considered.

In summary, the association between OMG and thymic hyperplasia and thymoma is close. These thymic lesions promote the release of self-reactive T cells and B cells by affecting the negative selection function of T cells and the activation state of B cells, thereby producing antibodies leading to the occurrence of OMG.

References

1. Koneczny I, Herbst R. Myasthenia gravis: pathogenic effects of autoantibodies on neuromuscular architecture. Cells. 2019;8(7) https://doi.org/10.3390/cells8070671.
2. Ruff RL, Lisak RP. Nature and action of antibodies in myasthenia gravis. Neurol Clin. 2018;36(2):275–91. https://doi.org/10.1016/j.ncl.2018.01.001.
3. Wood SJ, Slater CR. Safety factor at the neuromuscular junction. Prog Neurobiol. 2001;64(4):393–429. https://doi.org/10.1016/s0301-0082(00)00055-1.
4. Elmqvist D, Hofmann WW, Kugelberg J, et al. An electrophysiological investigation of neuromuscular transmission in myasthenia gravis. J Physiol. 1964;174(3):417–34. https://doi.org/10.1113/jphysiol.1964.sp007495.
5. Ruff RL, Lennon VA. How myasthenia gravis alters the safety factor for neuromuscular transmission. J Neuroimmunol. 2008;201-202:13–20. https://doi.org/10.1016/j.jneuroim.2008.04.038.
6. Sanders DB. The electrodiagnosis of myasthenia gravis. Ann N Y Acad Sci. 1987;505:539–56. https://doi.org/10.1111/j.1749-6632.1987.tb51322.x.
7. Nemazee D. Mechanisms of central tolerance for B cells. Nat Rev Immunol. 2017;17(5):281–94. https://doi.org/10.1038/nri.2017.19.

8. O'Hare M, Doughty C. Update on ocular myasthenia gravis. Semin Neurol. 2019;39(6):749–60. https://doi.org/10.1055/s-0039-1700527.
9. Halverson R, Torres RM, Pelanda R. Receptor editing is the main mechanism of B cell tolerance toward membrane antigens. Nat Immunol. 2004;5(6):645–50. https://doi.org/10.1038/ni1076.
10. Vander Heiden JA, Stathopoulos P, Zhou JQ, et al. Dysregulation of B cell repertoire formation in myasthenia gravis patients revealed through deep sequencing. J Immunol. 2017;198(4):1460–73. https://doi.org/10.4049/jimmunol.1601415.
11. Lee J-Y, Stathopoulos P, Gupta S, et al. Compromised fidelity of B-cell tolerance checkpoints in AChR and MuSK myasthenia gravis. Ann Clin Transl Neurol. 2016;3(6):443–54. https://doi.org/10.1002/acn3.311.
12. Evoli A, Caliandro P, Iorio R, et al. Poly-autoimmunity in patients with myasthenia gravis: a single-center experience. Autoimmunity. 2015;48(6):412–7. https://doi.org/10.3109/08916934.2015.1031890.
13. Bakhru P, Su MA. Estrogen turns down "the AIRE". J Clin Invest. 2016;126(4):1239–41. https://doi.org/10.1172/jci86800.
14. Dragin N, Bismuth J, Cizeron-Clairac G, et al. Estrogen-mediated downregulation of AIRE influences sexual dimorphism in autoimmune diseases. J Clin Invest. 2016;126(4):1525–37. https://doi.org/10.1172/jci81894.
15. Perry JSA, Lio CJ, Kau AL, et al. Distinct contributions of Aire and antigen-presenting-cell subsets to the generation of self-tolerance in the thymus. Immunity. 2014;41(3):414–26. https://doi.org/10.1016/j.immuni.2014.08.007.
16. Klein L, Kyewski B, Allen PM, et al. Positive and negative selection of the T cell repertoire: what thymocytes see (and don't see). Nat Rev Immunol. 2014;14(6):377–91. https://doi.org/10.1038/nri3667.
17. Marx A, Pfister F, Schalke B, et al. The different roles of the thymus in the pathogenesis of the various myasthenia gravis subtypes. Autoimmun Rev. 2013;12(9):875–84. https://doi.org/10.1016/j.autrev.2013.03.007.
18. Hohlfeld R, Toyka KV, Heininger K, et al. Autoimmune human T lymphocytes specific for acetylcholine receptor. Nature. 1984;310(5974):244–6. https://doi.org/10.1038/310244a0.
19. Nagvekar N, Moody AM, Moss P, et al. A pathogenetic role for the thymoma in myasthenia gravis. Autosensitization of IL-4- producing T cell clones recognizing extracellular acetylcholine receptor epitopes presented by minority class II isotypes. J Clin Invest. 1998;101(10):2268–77. https://doi.org/10.1172/jci2068.
20. Vrolix K, Fraussen J, Losen M, et al. Clonal heterogeneity of thymic B cells from early-onset myasthenia gravis patients with antibodies against the acetylcholine receptor. J Autoimmun. 2014;52:101–12. https://doi.org/10.1016/j.jaut.2013.12.008.
21. Marx A, Willcox N, Leite MI, et al. Thymoma and paraneoplastic myasthenia gravis. Autoimmunity. 2010;43(5-6):413–27. https://doi.org/10.3109/08916930903555935.
22. Buckley C, Douek D, Newsom-Davis J, et al. Mature, long-lived CD4+ and CD8+ T cells are generated by the thymoma in myasthenia gravis. Ann Neurol. 2001;50(1):64–72. https://doi.org/10.1002/ana.1017.
23. Song Y, Zhou L, Miao F, et al. Increased frequency of thymic T follicular helper cells in myasthenia gravis patients with thymoma. J Thorac Dis. 2016;8(3):314–22. https://doi.org/10.21037/jtd.2016.03.03.
24. Zhang X, Liu S, Chang T, et al. Intrathymic Tfh/B cells interaction leads to ectopic GCs formation and anti-AChR antibody production: central role in triggering MG occurrence. Mol Neurobiol. 2016;53(1):120–31. https://doi.org/10.1007/s12035-014-8985-1.
25. Steinman L. A brief history of T(H)17, the first major revision in the T(H)1/T(H)2 hypothesis of T cell-mediated tissue damage. Nat Med. 2007;13(2):139–45. https://doi.org/10.1038/nm1551.
26. Roche JC, Capablo JL, Larrad L, et al. Increased serum interleukin-17 levels in patients with myasthenia gravis. Muscle Nerve. 2011;44(2):278–80. https://doi.org/10.1002/mus.22070.
27. Wang Z, Wang W, Chen Y, et al. T helper type 17 cells expand in patients with myasthenia-associated thymoma. Scand J Immunol. 2012;76(1):54–61. https://doi.org/10.1111/j.1365-3083.2012.02703.x.
28. Yi JS, Guidon A, Sparks S, et al. Characterization of CD4 and CD8 T cell responses in MuSK myasthenia gravis. J Autoimmun. 2014;52:130–8. https://doi.org/10.1016/j.jaut.2013.12.005.
29. Schaffert H, Pelz A, Saxena A, et al. IL-17-producing CD4(+) T cells contribute to the loss of B-cell tolerance in experimental autoimmune myasthenia gravis. Eur J Immunol. 2015;45(5):1339–47. https://doi.org/10.1002/eji.201445064.
30. Thiruppathi M, Rowin J, Ganesh B, et al. Impaired regulatory function in circulating CD4(+)CD25(high)CD127(low/−) T cells in patients with myasthenia gravis. Clin Immunol. 2012;145(3):209–23. https://doi.org/10.1016/j.clim.2012.09.012.
31. Nishimura T, Inaba Y, Nakazawa Y, et al. Reduction in peripheral regulatory T cell population in childhood ocular type myasthenia gravis. Brain Dev. 2015;37(8):808–16. https://doi.org/10.1016/j.braindev.2014.12.007.
32. Luther C, Poeschel S, Varga M, et al. Decreased frequency of intrathymic regulatory T cells in patients with myasthenia-associated thymoma. J Neuroimmunol. 2005;164(1-2):124–8. https://doi.org/10.1016/j.jneuroim.2005.03.011.
33. Fattorossi A, Battaglia A, Buzzonetti A, et al. Thymopoiesis, regulatory T cells, and TCRVbeta expression in thymoma with and without myasthenia

gravis, and modulatory effects of steroid therapy. J Clin Immunol. 2008;28(2):194–206. https://doi.org/10.1007/s10875-007-9147-2.
34. Berrih-Aknin S, Le Panse R. Myasthenia gravis: a comprehensive review of immune dysregulation and etiological mechanisms. J Autoimmun. 2014;52:90–100. https://doi.org/10.1016/j.jaut.2013.12.011.
35. Trouth AJ, Dabi A, Solieman N, et al. Myasthenia gravis: a review. Autoimmune Dis. 2012;2012:874680. https://doi.org/10.1155/2012/874680.
36. Shen C, Lu Y, Zhang B, et al. Antibodies against low-density lipoprotein receptor-related protein 4 induce myasthenia gravis. J Clin Invest. 2013;123(12):5190–202. https://doi.org/10.1172/jci66039.
37. Del Castillo J, Katz B. On the localization of acetylcholine receptors. J Physiol. 1955;128(1):157–81. https://doi.org/10.1113/jphysiol.1955.sp005297.
38. Nickel E, Potter LT. Ultrastructure of isolated membranes of Torpedo electric tissue. Brain Res. 1973;57(2):508–17. https://doi.org/10.1016/0006-8993(73)90158-3.
39. Toyoshima C, Unwin N. Ion channel of acetylcholine receptor reconstructed from images of postsynaptic membranes. Nature. 1988;336(6196):247–50. https://doi.org/10.1038/336247a0.
40. Lindstrom JM. Acetylcholine receptors and myasthenia. Muscle Nerve. 2000;23(4):453–77. https://doi.org/10.1002/(sici)1097-4598(200004)23:4<453::aid-mus3>3.0.co;2-o.
41. Patrick J, Ballivet M, Boas L, et al. Molecular cloning of the acetylcholine receptor. Cold Spring Harb Symp Quant Biol. 1983;48(Pt 1):71–8. https://doi.org/10.1101/sqb.1983.048.01.009.
42. Luo J, Lindstrom J. Antigenic structure of the human muscle nicotinic acetylcholine receptor main immunogenic region. J Mol Neurosci. 2010;40(1-2):217–20. https://doi.org/10.1007/s12031-009-9271-y.
43. Kordas G, Lagoumintzis G, Sideris S, et al. Direct proof of the in vivo pathogenic role of the AChR autoantibodies from myasthenia gravis patients. PLoS One. 2014;9(9):e108327. https://doi.org/10.1371/journal.pone.0108327.
44. Saxena A, Stevens J, Cetin H, et al. Characterization of an anti-fetal AChR monoclonal antibody isolated from a myasthenia gravis patient. Sci Rep. 2017;7(1):14426. https://doi.org/10.1038/s41598-017-14350-8.
45. Makino T, Nakamura R, Terakawa M, et al. Analysis of peripheral B cells and autoantibodies against the anti-nicotinic acetylcholine receptor derived from patients with myasthenia gravis using single-cell manipulation tools. PLoS One. 2017;12(10):e0185976. https://doi.org/10.1371/journal.pone.0185976.
46. Gomez AM, Van Den Broeck J, Vrolix K, et al. Antibody effector mechanisms in myasthenia gravis-pathogenesis at the neuromuscular junction. Autoimmunity. 2010;43(5-6):353–70. https://doi.org/10.3109/08916930903555943.
47. Engel AG, Arahata K. The membrane attack complex of complement at the endplate in myasthenia gravis. Ann N Y Acad Sci. 1987;505:326–32. https://doi.org/10.1111/j.1749-6632.1987.tb51301.x.
48. Muppidi S, Utsugisawa K, Benatar M, et al. Long-term safety and efficacy of eculizumab in generalized myasthenia gravis. Muscle Nerve. 2019;60(1):14–24. https://doi.org/10.1002/mus.26447.
49. Drachman DB, Angus CW, Adams RN, et al. Myasthenic antibodies cross-link acetylcholine receptors to accelerate degradation. N Engl J Med. 1978;298(20):1116–22. https://doi.org/10.1056/nejm197805182982004.
50. Kang S-Y, Oh J-H, Song SK, et al. Both binding and blocking antibodies correlate with disease severity in myasthenia gravis. Neurol Sci. 2015;36(7):1167–71. https://doi.org/10.1007/s10072-015-2236-8.
51. Haven TR, Astill ME, Pasi BM, et al. An algorithm for acetylcholine receptor antibody testing in patients with suspected myasthenia gravis. Clin Chem. 2010;56(6):1028–9. https://doi.org/10.1373/clinchem.2009.140392.
52. Agius MA, Richman DP, Vincent A, et al. Autoantibody testing in the diagnosis and management of autoimmune disorders of neuromuscular transmission and related diseases. In: Myasthenia gravis and related disorders; 2009. p. 143–56.
53. Vernino S, Lennon VA. Autoantibody profiles and neurological correlations of thymoma. Clin Cancer Res. 2004;10(21):7270–5. https://doi.org/10.1158/1078-0432.Ccr-04-0735.
54. Cortes-Vicente E, Alvarez-Velasco R, Segovia S, et al. Clinical and therapeutic features of myasthenia gravis in adults based on age at onset. Neurology. 2020;94(11):E1171–80. https://doi.org/10.1212/wnl.0000000000008903.
55. Verschuuren JJ, Huijbers MG, Plomp JJ, et al. Pathophysiology of myasthenia gravis with antibodies to the acetylcholine receptor, muscle-specific kinase and low-density lipoprotein receptor-related protein 4. Autoimmun Rev. 2013;12(9):918–23. https://doi.org/10.1016/j.autrev.2013.03.001.
56. Oosterhuis HJ, Limburg PC, Hummel-Tappel E, et al. Anti-acetylcholine receptor antibodies in myasthenia gravis. Part 2. Clinical and serological follow-up of individual patients. J Neurol Sci. 1983;58(3):371–85. https://doi.org/10.1016/0022-510x(83)90096-5.
57. Bartoccioni E, Scuderi F, Minicuci GM, et al. Anti-MuSK antibodies: correlation with myasthenia gravis severity. Neurology. 2006;67(3):505–7.
58. Peeler CE, De Lott LB, Nagia L, et al. Clinical utility of acetylcholine receptor antibody testing in ocular myasthenia gravis. JAMA Neurol. 2015;72(10):1170–4. https://doi.org/10.1001/jamaneurol.2015.1444.
59. Feng X, Huan X, Yan C, et al. Adult ocular myasthenia gravis conversion: a single-center retrospective

analysis in China. Eur Neurol. 2020;83(2):182–8. https://doi.org/10.1159/000507853.
60. Supawongwattana M, Vanikieti K, Jindahra P, et al. Significance of acetylcholine receptor antibody titers in acetylcholine receptor antibody-positive ocular myasthenia gravis: generalization and presence of thyroid autoimmune antibodies and thymoma. Clin Ophthalmol. 2023;17:649–56. https://doi.org/10.2147/opth.S402181.
61. Lindstrom J. An assay for antibodies to human acetylcholine receptor in serum from patients with myasthenia gravis. Clin Immunol Immunopathol. 1977;7(1):36–43. https://doi.org/10.1016/0090-1229(77)90027-7.
62. Lazaridis K, Tzartos SJ. Autoantibody specificities in myasthenia gravis; implications for improved diagnostics and therapeutics. Front Immunol. 2020;11:212. https://doi.org/10.3389/fimmu.2020.00212.
63. Yang L, Maxwell S, Leite MI, et al. Non-radioactive serological diagnosis of myasthenia gravis and clinical features of patients from Tianjin, China. J Neurol Sci. 2011;301(1-2):71–6. https://doi.org/10.1016/j.jns.2010.10.023.
64. Cruz PMR, Al-Hajjar M, Huda S, et al. Clinical features and diagnostic usefulness of antibodies to clustered acetylcholine receptors in the diagnosis of seronegative myasthenia gravis. JAMA Neurol. 2015;72(6):642–9. https://doi.org/10.1001/jamaneurol.2015.0203.
65. Jacob S, Viegas S, Leite MI, et al. Presence and pathogenic relevance of antibodies to clustered acetylcholine receptor in ocular and generalized myasthenia gravis. Arch Neurol. 2012;69(8):994–1001. https://doi.org/10.1001/archneurol.2012.437.
66. Hoch W, McConville J, Helms S, et al. Autoantibodies to the receptor tyrosine kinase MuSK in patients with myasthenia gravis without acetylcholine receptor antibodies. Nat Med. 2001;7(3):365–8. https://doi.org/10.1038/85520.
67. Jennings CG, Dyer SM, Burden SJ. Muscle-specific trk-related receptor with a kringle domain defines a distinct class of receptor tyrosine kinases. Proc Natl Acad Sci U S A. 1993;90(7):2895–9. https://doi.org/10.1073/pnas.90.7.2895.
68. Valenzuela DM, Stitt TN, DiStefano PS, et al. Receptor tyrosine kinase specific for the skeletal muscle lineage: expression in embryonic muscle, at the neuromuscular junction, and after injury. Neuron. 1995;15(3):573–84. https://doi.org/10.1016/0896-6273(95)90146-9.
69. Garcia-Osta A, Tsokas P, Pollonini G, et al. MuSK expressed in the brain mediates cholinergic responses, synaptic plasticity, and memory formation. J Neurosci. 2006;26(30):7919–32. https://doi.org/10.1523/jneurosci.1674-06.2006.
70. Huijbers MG, Zhang W, Klooster R, et al. MuSK IgG4 autoantibodies cause myasthenia gravis by inhibiting binding between MuSK and Lrp4. Proc Natl Acad Sci U S A. 2013;110(51):20783–8. https://doi.org/10.1073/pnas.1313944110.
71. Koneczny I, Cossins J, Waters P, et al. MuSK myasthenia gravis IgG4 disrupts the interaction of LRP4 with MuSK but both IgG4 and IgG1-3 can disperse preformed agrin-independent AChR clusters. PLoS One. 2013;8(11):e80695. https://doi.org/10.1371/journal.pone.0080695.
72. Koneczny I, Stevens JA, De Rosa A, et al. IgG4 autoantibodies against muscle-specific kinase undergo Fab-arm exchange in myasthenia gravis patients. J Autoimmun. 2017;77:104–15. https://doi.org/10.1016/j.jaut.2016.11.005.
73. Mori S, Kubo S, Akiyoshi T, et al. Antibodies against muscle-specific kinase impair both presynaptic and postsynaptic functions in a murine model of myasthenia gravis. Am J Pathol. 2012;180(2):798–810. https://doi.org/10.1016/j.ajpath.2011.10.031.
74. Mori S, Yamada S, Kubo S, et al. Divalent and monovalent autoantibodies cause dysfunction of MuSK by distinct mechanisms in a rabbit model of myasthenia gravis. J Neuroimmunol. 2012;244(1-2):1–7. https://doi.org/10.1016/j.jneuroim.2011.12.005.
75. Klooster R, Plomp JJ, Huijbers MG, et al. Muscle-specific kinase myasthenia gravis IgG4 autoantibodies cause severe neuromuscular junction dysfunction in mice. Brain. 2012;135(Pt 4):1081–101. https://doi.org/10.1093/brain/aws025.
76. Kawakami Y, Ito M, Hirayama M, et al. Anti-MuSK autoantibodies block binding of collagen Q to MuSK. Neurology. 2011;77(20):1819–26. https://doi.org/10.1212/WNL.0b013e318237f660.
77. Hatanaka Y, Hemmi S, Morgan M, et al. Nonresponsiveness to anticholinesterase agents in patients with MuSK-antibody-positive MG. Neurology. 2005;65:1508–9.
78. Kostera-Pruszczyk A, Kamińska A, Dutkiewicz M, et al. MuSK-positive myasthenia gravis is rare in the Polish population. Eur J Neurol. 2008;15(7):720–4. https://doi.org/10.1111/j.1468-1331.2008.02176.x.
79. Leite MI, Jacob S, Viegas S, et al. IgG1 antibodies to acetylcholine receptors in 'seronegative' myasthenia gravis. Brain. 2008;131(Pt 7):1940–52. https://doi.org/10.1093/brain/awn092.
80. Muppidi S, Wolfe GI. Muscle-specific receptor tyrosine kinase antibody-positive and seronegative myasthenia gravis. Front Neurol Neurosci. 2009;26:109–19. https://doi.org/10.1159/000212372.
81. Tsonis AI, Zisimopoulou P, Lazaridis K, et al. MuSK autoantibodies in myasthenia gravis detected by cell based assay—a multinational study. J Neuroimmunol. 2015;284:10–7. https://doi.org/10.1016/j.jneuroim.2015.04.015.
82. Suzuki S, Utsugisawa K, Nagane Y, et al. Clinical and immunological differences between early and late-onset myasthenia gravis in Japan. J Neuroimmunol. 2011;230(1-2):148–52. https://doi.org/10.1016/j.jneuroim.2010.10.023.

83. Luther C, Adamopoulou E, Stoeckle C, et al. Prednisolone treatment induces tolerogenic dendritic cells and a regulatory milieu in myasthenia gravis patients. J Immunol. 2009;183(2):841–8. https://doi.org/10.4049/jimmunol.0802046.
84. Wu B, Wan Y. Molecular control of pathogenic Th17 cells in autoimmune diseases. Int Immunopharmacol. 2020;80:106187. https://doi.org/10.1016/j.intimp.2020.106187.
85. Han J, Zhang J, Li M, et al. A novel MuSK cell-based myasthenia gravis diagnostic assay. J Neuroimmunol. 2019;337:577076. https://doi.org/10.1016/j.jneuroim.2019.577076.
86. Wu B, Zhang S, Guo Z, et al. The TGF-β superfamily cytokine Activin-A is induced during autoimmune neuroinflammation and drives pathogenic Th17 cell differentiation. Immunity. 2021;54(2):308–323.e306. https://doi.org/10.1016/j.immuni.2020.12.010.
87. Souroujon MC, Aricha R, Feferman T, et al. Regulatory T cell-based immunotherapies in experimental autoimmune myasthenia gravis. Ann N Y Acad Sci. 2012;1274:120–6. https://doi.org/10.1111/j.1749-6632.2012.06844.x.
88. Ohta K, Shigemoto K, Kubo S, et al. MuSK antibodies in AChR Ab-seropositive MG vs AChR Ab-seronegative MG. Neurology. 2004;62(11):2132–3. https://doi.org/10.1212/01.wnl.0000129274.12702.92.
89. Niks EH, van Leeuwen Y, Leite MI, et al. Clinical fluctuations in MuSK myasthenia gravis are related to antigen-specific IgG4 instead of IgG1. J Neuroimmunol. 2008;195(1-2):151–6. https://doi.org/10.1016/j.jneuroim.2008.01.013.
90. Mantegazza R, Antozzi C. When myasthenia gravis is deemed refractory: clinical signposts and treatment strategies. Ther Adv Neurol Disord. 2018;11:1756285617749134. https://doi.org/10.1177/1756285617749134.
91. Guptill JT, Sanders DB, Evoli A. Anti-musk antibody myasthenia gravis: clinical findings and response to treatment in two large cohorts. Muscle Nerve. 2011;44(1):36–40. https://doi.org/10.1002/mus.22006.
92. Matthews I, Chen S, Hewer R, et al. Muscle-specific receptor tyrosine kinase autoantibodies—a new immunoprecipitation assay. Clin Chim Acta. 2004;348(1-2):95–9. https://doi.org/10.1016/j.cccn.2004.05.008.
93. Vincent A, Newsom-Davis J. Acetylcholine receptor antibody as a diagnostic test for myasthenia gravis: results in 153 validated cases and 2967 diagnostic assays. J Neurol Neurosurg Psychiatry. 1985;48(12):1246–52. https://doi.org/10.1136/jnnp.48.12.1246.
94. Trakas N, Zisimopoulou P, Tzartos SJ. Development of a highly sensitive diagnostic assay for muscle-specific tyrosine kinase (MuSK) autoantibodies in myasthenia gravis. J Neuroimmunol. 2011;240-241:79–86. https://doi.org/10.1016/j.jneuroim.2011.09.007.
95. Guptill JT, Yi JS, Sanders DB, et al. Characterization of B cells in muscle-specific kinase antibody myasthenia gravis. Neurol Neuroimmunol Neuroinflamm. 2015;2(2):e77. https://doi.org/10.1212/nxi.0000000000000077.
96. Tüzün E, Christadoss P. Complement associated pathogenic mechanisms in myasthenia gravis. Autoimmun Rev. 2013;12(9):904–11. https://doi.org/10.1016/j.autrev.2013.03.003.
97. Chang T, Leite MI, Senanayake S, et al. Clinical and serological study of myasthenia gravis using both radioimmunoprecipitation and cell-based assays in a South Asian population. J Neurol Sci. 2014;343(1-2):82–7. https://doi.org/10.1016/j.jns.2014.05.037.
98. Park KH, Waters P, Woodhall M, et al. Myasthenia gravis seronegative for acetylcholine receptor antibodies in South Korea: autoantibody profiles and clinical features. PLoS One. 2018;13(3):e0193723. https://doi.org/10.1371/journal.pone.0193723.
99. Tsujihata M, Yoshimura T, Satoh A, et al. Diagnostic significance of IgG, C3, and C9 at the limb muscle motor end-plate in minimal myasthenia gravis. Neurology. 1989;39(10):1359–63. https://doi.org/10.1212/wnl.39.10.1359.
100. Kim N, Stiegler A, Cameron TO, et al. Lrp4 is a receptor for Agrin and forms a complex with MuSK. Cell. 2008;135(2):334–42. https://doi.org/10.1016/j.cell.2008.10.002.
101. Zhang W, Coldefy AS, Hubbard SR, et al. Agrin binds to the N-terminal region of Lrp4 protein and stimulates association between Lrp4 and the first immunoglobulin-like domain in muscle-specific kinase (MuSK). J Biol Chem. 2011;286(47):40624–30. https://doi.org/10.1074/jbc.M111.279307.
102. Bacchi S, Kramer P, Chalk C. Autoantibodies to low-density lipoprotein receptor-related protein 4 in double seronegative myasthenia gravis: a systematic review. Can J Neurol Sci. 2018;45(1):62–7. https://doi.org/10.1017/cjn.2017.253.
103. Pevzner A, Schoser B, Peters K, et al. Anti-LRP4 autoantibodies in AChR- and MuSK-antibody-negative myasthenia gravis. J Neurol. 2012;259(3):427–35. https://doi.org/10.1007/s00415-011-6194-7.
104. Higuchi O, Hamuro J, Motomura M, et al. Autoantibodies to low-density lipoprotein receptor-related protein 4 in myasthenia gravis. Ann Neurol. 2011;69(2):418–22. https://doi.org/10.1002/ana.22312.
105. Zhang B, Tzartos JS, Belimezi M, et al. Autoantibodies to lipoprotein-related protein 4 in patients with double-seronegative myasthenia gravis. Arch Neurol. 2012;69(4):445–51. https://doi.org/10.1001/archneurol.2011.2393.
106. Zisimopoulou P, Evangelakou P, Tzartos J, et al. A comprehensive analysis of the epidemiology and

clinical characteristics of anti-LRP4 in myasthenia gravis. J Autoimmun. 2014;52:139–45. https://doi.org/10.1016/j.jaut.2013.12.004.
107. Li M, Han J, Zhang Y, et al. Clinical analysis of Chinese anti-low-density-lipoprotein-receptor--associated protein 4 antibodies in patients with myasthenia gravis. Eur J Neurol. 2019;26(10):1296–1.e1284. https://doi.org/10.1111/ene.13979.
108. Li Y, Zhang Y, Cai G, et al. Anti-LRP4 autoantibodies in Chinese patients with myasthenia gravis. Muscle Nerve. 2017;56(5):938–42. https://doi.org/10.1002/mus.25591.
109. Cordts I, Bodart N, Hartmann K, et al. Screening for lipoprotein receptor-related protein 4-, agrin-, and titin-antibodies and exploring the autoimmune spectrum in myasthenia gravis. J Neurol. 2017;264(6):1193–203. https://doi.org/10.1007/s00415-017-8514-z.
110. Tzartos JS, Zisimopoulou P, Rentzos M, et al. LRP4 antibodies in serum and CSF from amyotrophic lateral sclerosis patients. Ann Clin Transl Neurol. 2014;1(2):80–7. https://doi.org/10.1002/acn3.26.
111. Rivner MH, Liu S, Quarles B, et al. Agrin and low-density lipoprotein-related receptor protein 4 antibodies in amyotrophic lateral sclerosis patients. Muscle Nerve. 2017;55(3):430–2. https://doi.org/10.1002/mus.25438.
112. Hoshi T, Tezuka T, Yokoyama K, et al. Mesdc2 plays a key role in cell-surface expression of Lrp4 and postsynaptic specialization in myotubes. FEBS Lett. 2013;587(23):3749–54. https://doi.org/10.1016/j.febslet.2013.10.001.
113. Dalakas MC. Role of complement, anti-complement therapeutics, and other targeted immunotherapies in myasthenia gravis. Expert Rev Clin Immunol. 2022;18(7):691–701. https://doi.org/10.1080/1744666x.2022.2082946.
114. Stathopoulos P, Kumar A, Heiden JAV, et al. Mechanisms underlying B cell immune dysregulation and autoantibody production in MuSK myasthenia gravis. Ann N Y Acad Sci. 2018;1412(1):154–65. https://doi.org/10.1111/nyas.13535.
115. Uzawa A, Kuwabara S, Suzuki S, et al. Roles of cytokines and T cells in the pathogenesis of myasthenia gravis. Clin Exp Immunol. 2021;203(3):366–74. https://doi.org/10.1111/cei.13546.
116. Sudres M, Verdier J, Truffault F, et al. Pathophysiological mechanisms of autoimmunity. Ann N Y Acad Sci. 2018;1413(1):59–68. https://doi.org/10.1111/nyas.13560.
117. Dominguez-Villar M, Hafler DA. Regulatory T cells in autoimmune disease. Nat Immunol. 2018;19(7):665–73. https://doi.org/10.1038/s41590-018-0120-4.
118. Aguilo-Seara G, Xie Y, Sheehan J, et al. Ablation of IL-17 expression moderates experimental autoimmune myasthenia gravis disease severity. Cytokine. 2017;96:279–85. https://doi.org/10.1016/j.cyto.2017.05.008.
119. Yi JS, Guptill JT, Stathopoulos P, et al. B cells in the pathophysiology of myasthenia gravis. Muscle Nerve. 2018;57(2):172–84. https://doi.org/10.1002/mus.25973.
120. Veldhoen M, Hocking RJ, Atkins CJ, et al. TGFbeta in the context of an inflammatory cytokine milieu supports de novo differentiation of IL-17-producing T cells. Immunity. 2006;24(2):179–89. https://doi.org/10.1016/j.immuni.2006.01.001.
121. Lu L, Barbi J, Pan F. The regulation of immune tolerance by FOXP3. Nat Rev Immunol. 2017;17(11):703–17. https://doi.org/10.1038/nri.2017.75.
122. Fattorossi A, Battaglia A, Buzzonetti A, et al. Circulating and thymic CD4 CD25 T regulatory cells in myasthenia gravis: effect of immunosuppressive treatment. Immunology. 2005;116(1):134–41. https://doi.org/10.1111/j.1365-2567.2005.02220.x.
123. Aricha R, Feferman T, Fuchs S, et al. Ex vivo generated regulatory T cells modulate experimental autoimmune myasthenia gravis. J Immunol. 2008;180(4):2132–9. https://doi.org/10.4049/jimmunol.180.4.2132.
124. Xu W, Ren M, Ghosh S, et al. Defects of CTLA-4 are associated with regulatory T cells in myasthenia gravis implicated by intravenous immunoglobulin therapy. Mediat Inflamm. 2020;2020:3645157. https://doi.org/10.1155/2020/3645157.
125. Gradolatto A, Nazzal D, Truffault F, et al. Both Treg cells and Tconv cells are defective in the Myasthenia gravis thymus: roles of IL-17 and TNF-α. J Autoimmun. 2014;52:53–63. https://doi.org/10.1016/j.jaut.2013.12.015.
126. Jonsson DI, Pirskanen R, Piehl F. Beneficial effect of tocilizumab in myasthenia gravis refractory to rituximab. Neuromuscul Disord. 2017;27(6):565–8. https://doi.org/10.1016/j.nmd.2017.03.007.
127. Beecher G, Putko BN, Wagner AN, et al. Therapies directed against B-cells and downstream effectors in generalized autoimmune myasthenia gravis: current status. Drugs. 2019;79(4):353–64. https://doi.org/10.1007/s40265-019-1065-0.
128. Gabrilovich DI, Nagaraj S. Myeloid-derived suppressor cells as regulators of the immune system. Nat Rev Immunol. 2009;9(3):162–74. https://doi.org/10.1038/nri2506.
129. Marvel D, Gabrilovich DI. Myeloid-derived suppressor cells in the tumor microenvironment: expect the unexpected. J Clin Invest. 2015;125(9):3356–64. https://doi.org/10.1172/jci80005.
130. Tedder TF. B10 cells: a functionally defined regulatory B cell subset. J Immunol. 2015;194(4):1395–401. https://doi.org/10.4049/jimmunol.1401329.
131. Sun F, Ladha SS, Yang L, et al. Interleukin-10 producing-B cells and their association with responsiveness to rituximab in myasthenia gravis. Muscle Nerve. 2014;49(4):487–94. https://doi.org/10.1002/mus.23951.

132. Gilhus N, Skeie G, Romi F, et al. Myasthenia gravis—autoantibody characteristics and their implications for therapy. Nat Rev Neurol. 2016;12(5):259–68. https://doi.org/10.1038/nrneurol.2016.44.
133. Romi F, Kristoffersen EK, Aarli JA, et al. The role of complement in myasthenia gravis: serological evidence of complement consumption in vivo. J Neuroimmunol. 2005;158(1-2):191–4. https://doi.org/10.1016/j.jneuroim.2004.08.002.
134. Yang H, Wu B, Tüzün E, et al. A new mouse model of autoimmune ocular myasthenia gravis. Invest Ophthalmol Vis Sci. 2007;48(11):5101–11. https://doi.org/10.1167/iovs.07-0271.
135. Wu X, Tuzun E, Saini SS, et al. Ocular myasthenia gravis induced by human acetylcholine receptor ϵ subunit immunization in HLA DR3 transgenic mice. Immunol Lett. 2015;168(2):306–12. https://doi.org/10.1016/j.imlet.2015.10.009.
136. Wu X, Tuzun E, Li J, et al. Ocular and generalized myasthenia gravis induced by human acetylcholine receptor γ subunit immunization. Muscle Nerve. 2012;45(2):209–16. https://doi.org/10.1002/mus.22273.
137. Soltys J, Gong B, Kaminski HJ, et al. Extraocular muscle susceptibility to myasthenia gravis: unique immunological environment? Ann N Y Acad Sci. 2008;1132:220–4. https://doi.org/10.1196/annals.1405.037.
138. JF H Jr. Myasthenia gravis: the role of complement at the neuromuscular junction. Ann N Y Acad Sci. 2018;1412(1):113–28. https://doi.org/10.1111/nyas.13522.
139. Liu A, Lin H, Liu Y, et al. Correlation of C3 level with severity of generalized myasthenia gravis. Muscle Nerve. 2009;40(5):801–8. https://doi.org/10.1002/mus.21398.
140. Marx A, Muller-Hermelink HK, Strobel P. The role of thymomas in the development of myasthenia gravis. In: Agius MA, Richman DP, Fairclough RH, et al., editors. Myasthenia gravis and related disorders: biochemical basis for disease of the neuromuscular junction; 2003. p. 223–36.
141. Wang HX, Pan W, Zheng L, et al. Thymic epithelial cells contribute to thymopoiesis and T cell development. Front Immunol. 2019;10:3099. https://doi.org/10.3389/fimmu.2019.03099.
142. Takaba H, Takayanagi H. The mechanisms of T cell selection in the thymus. Trends Immunol. 2017;38(11):805–16. https://doi.org/10.1016/j.it.2017.07.010.
143. Poëa-Guyon S, Christadoss P, Le Panse R, et al. Effects of cytokines on acetylcholine receptor expression: implications for myasthenia gravis. J Immunol (Baltimore, MD: 1950). 2005;174(10):5941–9.
144. Ströbel P, Murumägi A, Klein R, et al. Deficiency of the autoimmune regulator AIRE in thymomas is insufficient to elicit autoimmune polyendocrinopathy syndrome type 1 (APS-1). J Pathol. 2007;211(5):563–71. https://doi.org/10.1002/path.2141.
145. Liu Y, Zhang H, Zhang P, et al. Autoimmune regulator expression in thymomas with or without autoimmune disease. Immunol Lett. 2014;161(1):50–6. https://doi.org/10.1016/j.imlet.2014.04.008.
146. Berrih-Aknin S, Panse RL, Dragin N. AIRE: a missing link to explain female susceptibility to autoimmune diseases. Ann N Y Acad Sci. 2018;1412(1):21–32. https://doi.org/10.1111/nyas.13529.
147. Kohler S, Keil TO, Swierzy M, et al. Disturbed B cell subpopulations and increased plasma cells in myasthenia gravis patients. J Neuroimmunol. 2013;264(1-2):114–9. https://doi.org/10.1016/j.jneuroim.2013.09.006.
148. Honnorat J, Antoine JC. Paraneoplastic neurological syndromes. Orphanet J Rare Dis. 2007;2:22. https://doi.org/10.1186/1750-1172-2-22.
149. Truffault F, de Montpreville V, Eymard B, et al. Thymic germinal centers and corticosteroids in myasthenia gravis: an immunopathological study in 1035 cases and a critical review. Clin Rev Allergy Immunol. 2017;52(1):108–24. https://doi.org/10.1007/s12016-016-8558-3.
150. Zaĭrat'iants OV. Thymus hyperplasia: classification, problems of patho- and morphogenesis, importance in human pathology. Arkh Patol. 1991;53(10):3–12.
151. Kee HJ, Yang HK, Hwang JM, et al. Evaluation and validation of sustained upgaze combined with the ice-pack test for ocular myasthenia gravis in Asians. Neuromuscul Disord. 2019;29(4):296–301. https://doi.org/10.1016/j.nmd.2018.12.011.
152. Priola AM, Priola SM. Imaging of thymus in myasthenia gravis: from thymic hyperplasia to thymic tumor. Clin Radiol. 2014;69(5):e230–45. https://doi.org/10.1016/j.crad.2014.01.005.
153. Leite MI, Jones M, Ströbel P, et al. Myasthenia gravis thymus: complement vulnerability of epithelial and myoid cells, complement attack on them, and correlations with autoantibody status. Am J Pathol. 2007;171(3):893–905. https://doi.org/10.2353/ajpath.2007.070240.
154. Sims GP, Shiono H, Willcox N, et al. Somatic hypermutation and selection of B cells in thymic germinal centers responding to acetylcholine receptor in myasthenia gravis. J Immunol. 2001;167(4):1935–44. https://doi.org/10.4049/jimmunol.167.4.1935.
155. Leprince C, Cohen-Kaminsky S, Berrih-Aknin S, et al. Thymic B cells from myasthenia gravis patients are activated B cells. Phenotypic and functional analysis. J Immunol. 1990;145(7):2115–22.
156. Shiono H, Roxanis I, Zhang W, et al. Scenarios for autoimmunization of T and B cells in myasthenia gravis. In: Agius MA, Richman DP, Fairclough RH, et al., editors. Myasthenia gravis and related disorders: biochemical basis for disease of the neuromuscular junction; 2003. p. 237–56.
157. Hill ME, Shiono H, Newsom-Davis J, et al. The myasthenia gravis thymus: a rare source of human autoantibody-secreting plasma cells for

testing potential therapeutics. J Neuroimmunol. 2008;201-202:50–6. https://doi.org/10.1016/j.jneuroim.2008.06.027.
158. Scadding GK, Vincent A, Newsom-Davis J, et al. Acetylcholine receptor antibody synthesis by thymic lymphocytes: correlation with thymic histology. Neurology. 1981;31(8):935–43. https://doi.org/10.1212/wnl.31.8.935.
159. Yamada Y, Weis CA, Thelen J, et al. Thymoma associated myasthenia gravis (TAMG): differential expression of functional pathways in relation to MG status in different thymoma histotypes. Front Immunol. 2020;11:664. https://doi.org/10.3389/fimmu.2020.00664.
160. Gilhus N, Tzartos S, Evoli A, et al. Myasthenia gravis. Nat Rev Dis Primers. 2019;5(1):30. https://doi.org/10.1038/s41572-019-0079-y.
161. Li H, Ruan Z, Gao F, et al. Thymectomy and risk of generalization in patients with ocular myasthenia gravis: a multicenter retrospective cohort study. Neurotherapeutics. 2021;18(4):2449–57. https://doi.org/10.1007/s13311-021-01129-z.
162. Shrager JB, Deeb ME, Mick R, et al. Transcervical thymectomy for myasthenia gravis achieves results comparable to thymectomy by sternotomy. Ann Thorac Surg. 2002;74(2):320–6.; discussion 326–327. https://doi.org/10.1016/s0003-4975(02)03722-0.
163. Sussman J, Farrugia ME, Maddison P, et al. Myasthenia gravis: association of British neurologists' management guidelines. Pract Neurol. 2015;15(3):199–206. https://doi.org/10.1136/practneurol-2015-001126.
164. Kaufman AJ, Palatt J, Sivak M, et al. Thymectomy for myasthenia gravis: complete stable remission and associated prognostic factors in over 1000 cases. Semin Thorac Cardiovasc Surg. 2016;28(2):561–8. https://doi.org/10.1053/j.semtcvs.2016.04.002.
165. Yu S, Li F, Chen B, et al. Eight-year follow-up of patients with myasthenia gravis after thymectomy. Acta Neurol Scand. 2015;131(2):94–101. https://doi.org/10.1111/ane.12289.
166. Newsom-Davis J, Willcox N, Scadding G, et al. Anti-acetylcholine receptor antibody synthesis by cultured lymphocytes in myasthenia gravis: thymic and peripheral blood cell interactions. Ann N Y Acad Sci. 1981;377:393–402. https://doi.org/10.1111/j.1749-6632.1981.tb33747.x.
167. Fujii Y, Monden Y, Hashimoto J, et al. Acetylcholine receptor antibody-producing cells in thymus and lymph nodes in myasthenia gravis. Clin Immunol Immunopathol. 1985;34(1):141–6. https://doi.org/10.1016/0090-1229(85)90018-2.
168. Fujii Y, Monden Y, Hashimoto J, et al. Acetylcholine receptor antibody production by bone marrow cells in a patient with myasthenia gravis. Neurology. 1985;35(4):577–9. https://doi.org/10.1212/wnl.35.4.577.
169. Fujii Y, Hashimoto J, Monden Y, et al. Specific activation of lymphocytes against acetylcholine receptor in the thymus in myasthenia gravis. J Immunol. 1986;136(3):887–91.
170. Fichtner ML, Jiang R, Bourke A, et al. Autoimmune pathology in myasthenia gravis disease subtypes is governed by divergent mechanisms of immunopathology. Front Immunol. 2020;11:776. https://doi.org/10.3389/fimmu.2020.00776.

3 Characteristics of Extraocular Muscles in Ocular Myasthenia Gravis

3.1 Inherent Characteristics of Extraocular Muscles Increase the Risk of Neuromuscular Transmission Disorders

Unlike other skeletal muscles, extraocular muscles express embryonic type AChR subtypes and adult type AChR subtypes, which indicates that the antigen target is only expressed at the neuromuscular junction in the eye can explain the autoimmune attack causing pure ocular muscle damage [1]. Autoantibodies targeting embryonic receptors do not seem to explain differential damage, a more likely explanation is that the intrinsic characteristics of extraocular muscles increase the risk of neuromuscular transmission disorders in extraocular muscles: (1) Extraocular muscles have immature synaptic folds and lower AChR density, which reduces the end-plate potential, thereby reducing the safety factor of neuromuscular transmission. (2) The extremely high frequency of motor neuron stimulation may make the synapses of extraocular muscles more prone to neuromuscular transmission disorders [2, 3]. (3) Over 20% of extraocular muscle fibers have neuromuscular junctions that support rigid muscle contraction rather than twitch muscle contraction. The contraction of rigid fibers highly depends on the amplitude of the end-plate potential, and the reduction in the amplitude of the end-plate potential caused by the loss of AChR will weaken the contraction force. (4) Endogenous complement regulatory factors can protect the postsynaptic surface at the neuromuscular junction from complement-mediated damage. Compared with other muscles, these regulatory factors are expressed at lower levels at the neuromuscular junctions of extraocular muscles [4, 5], making the neuromuscular junctions of extraocular muscles more susceptible to complement-mediated MG damage.

In non-ocular muscles, regardless of the subtype of pathogenic antibodies, the substantial structure of muscle fibers will change, leading to functional denervation, mainly type II fiber atrophy. In both AChR-Ab positive MG and MuSK-Ab positive MG, there is varying degrees of mitochondrial stress and damage. Type II fibers contain fewer mitochondria than type I fibers, which may explain the increased sensitivity of type II fibers to mitochondrial stress effects [6]. Compared with limb muscles, extraocular muscles show similar pathological features, but more severe. However, the few existing reports are based on muscle biopsies of extraocular muscles with severe ocular myasthenia and limb muscles with mild myasthenia. The pathological features of extraocular muscles are not unique to OMG, and this pathological situation can also exist in extraocular muscle paralysis caused by other reasons. The limb muscle biopsy of patients with chronic neurogenic myasthenia (such as spinal muscular atrophy) shows similar light microscope

Q. Zhou, J. Chen, *Ocular Myasthenia Gravis*, Experts' Perspectives on Medical Advances,
https://doi.org/10.1007/978-981-96-1245-1_3

and mitochondrial degenerative changes [7, 8], indicating that at least some of the features observed in myasthenia biopsies are nonspecific and related to denervation and poor contractility.

3.2 Unique Metabolic Characteristics of Extraocular Muscles such as High Frequency of Nerve Stimulation and High Energy Demand

In the experimental autoimmune myasthenia gravis animal model with AChR-Ab positivity, the biggest difference in transcription between extraocular muscles and limb muscles is the metabolic-related gene pathway, especially the transition to oxidative metabolism. The unique metabolic characteristics of extraocular muscles, such as high frequency of nerve stimulation and high energy demand, make extraocular muscles particularly susceptible to the effects of "MG-induced" oxidative metabolism and increased muscle protein hydrolysis, thereby reducing muscle strength generation [9]. Insufficient muscle strength generation will further affect the production of mitochondria [10], leading to muscle atrophy [11, 12].

3.3 The Response of Extraocular Muscles to Botulinum Toxin and Certain Growth Factors Is Different from that of Limb Skeletal Muscles

The response of extraocular muscles to botulinum toxin and certain growth factors is also different from that of limb skeletal muscles [13]. For example, chick embryos undergoing presynaptic "denervation" with botulinum toxin show severe limb muscle atrophy and almost complete fat replacement [14]; however, extraocular muscles injected with botulinum toxin, although temporarily paralyzed, do not show muscle atrophy. This phenomenon can explain the potential for continuous activation and reconstruction of extraocular muscle satellite cells [13, 15]. However, a single injection of specific muscle growth factors (BMP4, TGFB1, Wnt3A) into the extraocular muscles of mice resulted in a significant reduction in muscle strength and muscle fiber diameter when measured 7 days later [16]. Multiple results from animal models and in vitro C2C12 myotube cyclic stretching experiments suggest that preventing muscle/myotube from generating force for ≥48 h (compared to continuous stretching) will lead to changes in downstream transcription signals and muscle fiber atrophy. Extraocular muscles may be more susceptible to the influence of certain growth factors [17].

3.4 Changes in the IGF1 Signaling Pathway May Be One of the Effect Pathways in the Pathogenesis of Ocular Myasthenia Gravis Paralysis

At the molecular level, the significant reduction in muscle strength is promoted by downregulating the IGF1/Akt signaling pathway to promote muscle atrophy, while the IGF1/Akt signaling pathway usually produces a synthetic metabolic effect in muscles by inhibiting protein degradation and promoting protein synthesis [14]. Downregulation of key genes in the IGF1/Akt/mTOR signaling pathway has a negative impact on muscle contractile force and mitochondrial production [17]. This pathway is related to the pathogenesis of MG. The gene expression profile of transdifferentiated cardiomyocytes stimulated by MG serum shows that the high expression of IGF1R, AKT1, and AKT2 genes in the muscle cells of patients with drug-resistant ocular muscle paralysis is related compared to the MG control group (the group of extraocular muscles responsive to treatment) [18]. This suggests that changes in the IGF1 signaling pathway may be one of the effector pathways in the pathogenesis of MG extraocular muscle paralysis, but this still needs to be verified.

3.5 Dysfunctional Mitochondria Can Trigger Atrophy Signaling Pathways by Overproducing Reactive Oxygen Species

The histology of MG muscles shows that the mitochondrial homeostasis of mild myasthenia gravis muscles can also be affected. Chronic denervation has been shown to affect mitochondrial production [19], but within 7 days of denervation, there were significant changes in the muscle transcriptome, and mitochondrial homeostasis shifted from fusion to division and fragmentation [19, 20]. Dysfunctional mitochondria can further trigger the atrophy signaling pathway by overproducing reactive oxygen species.

3.6 The Reasons for the Susceptibility of the Levator Palpebrae Superioris Are Still Unclear

The reasons for the susceptibility of the levator palpebrae superioris are still unclear. When the eyelid is open, the levator palpebrae superioris is in a state of repeated activation, which may make it prone to conduction fatigue. The levator palpebrae superioris contains anti-fatigue muscle fiber types similar to those of the extraocular muscles, but it is currently unclear whether the connection anatomy of the levator palpebrae superioris has the susceptibility characteristics of neuromuscular transmission damage.

References

1. Wakkach A, Guyon T, Bruand C, et al. Expression of acetylcholine receptor genes in human thymic epithelial cells—implications for myasthenia gravis. J Immunol. 1996;157(8):3752–60.
2. Kaminski HJ, Li Z, Richmonds C, et al. Susceptibility of ocular tissues to autoimmune diseases. Ann N Y Acad Sci. 2003;998:362–74. https://doi.org/10.1196/annals.1254.043.
3. Kaminski HJ, Maas E, Spiegel P, et al. Why are eye muscles frequently involved in myasthenia gravis? Neurology. 1990;40(11):1663–9. https://doi.org/10.1212/wnl.40.11.1663.
4. Grob D, Brunner N, Namba T, et al. Lifetime course of myasthenia gravis. Muscle Nerve. 2008;37(2):141–9. https://doi.org/10.1002/mus.20950.
5. Gilhus N, Skeie G, Romi F, et al. Myasthenia gravis—autoantibody characteristics and their implications for therapy. Nat Rev Neurol. 2016;12(5):259–68. https://doi.org/10.1038/nrneurol.2016.44.
6. McKelvie P, Satchi K, McNab AA, et al. Orbicularis oculi: morphological changes mimicking mitochondrial cytopathy in a series of control normal muscles. Clin Experiment Ophthalmol. 2012;40(5):497–502. https://doi.org/10.1111/j.1442-9071.2011.02727.x.
7. Cenacchi G, Papa V, Fanin M, et al. Comparison of muscle ultrastructure in myasthenia gravis with anti-MuSK and anti-AChR antibodies. J Neurol. 2011;258(5):746–52. https://doi.org/10.1007/s00415-010-5823-x.
8. Borgia D, Malena A, Spinazzi M, et al. Increased mitophagy in the skeletal muscle of spinal and bulbar muscular atrophy patients. Hum Mol Genet. 2017;26(6):1087–103. https://doi.org/10.1093/hmg/ddx019.
9. Kaminski HJ, Himuro K, Alshaikh J, et al. Differential RNA expression profile of skeletal muscle induced by experimental autoimmune myasthenia gravis in rats. Front Physiol. 2016;7:524. https://doi.org/10.3389/fphys.2016.00524.
10. Andrade FH, McMullen CA, Rumbaut RE. Mitochondria are fast Ca2+ sinks in rat extraocular muscles: a novel regulatory influence on contractile function and metabolism. Invest Ophthalmol Vis Sci. 2005;46(12):4541–7. https://doi.org/10.1167/iovs.05-0809.
11. Patel SP, Gamboa JL, McMullen CA, et al. Lower respiratory capacity in extraocular muscle mitochondria: evidence for intrinsic differences in mitochondrial composition and function. Invest Ophthalmol Vis Sci. 2009;50(1):180–6. https://doi.org/10.1167/iovs.08-1911.
12. Yu Wai Man CY, Chinnery PF, Griffiths PG. Extraocular muscles have fundamentally distinct properties that make them selectively vulnerable to certain disorders. Neuromuscul Disord. 2005;15(1):17–23. https://doi.org/10.1016/j.nmd.2004.10.002.
13. Ugalde I, Christiansen SP, McLoon LK. Botulinum toxin treatment of extraocular muscles in rabbits results in increased myofiber remodeling. Invest Ophthalmol Vis Sci. 2005;46(11):4114–20. https://doi.org/10.1167/iovs.05-0549.
14. Schiaffino S, Mammucari C. Regulation of skeletal muscle growth by the IGF1-Akt/PKB pathway: insights from genetic models. Skelet Muscle. 2011;1(1):4. https://doi.org/10.1186/2044-5040-1-4.
15. Verma M, Fitzpatrick K, McLoon LK. Extraocular muscle repair and regeneration. Curr Ophthalmol Rep. 2017;5(3):207–15. https://doi.org/10.1007/s40135-017-0141-4.

16. Anderson BC, Christiansen SP, McLoon LK. Myogenic growth factors can decrease extraocular muscle force generation: a potential biological approach to the treatment of strabismus. Invest Ophthalmol Vis Sci. 2008;49(1):221–9. https://doi.org/10.1167/iovs.07-0600.
17. Soltow QA, Zeanah EH, Lira VA, et al. Cessation of cyclic stretch induces atrophy of C2C12 myotubes. Biochem Biophys Res Commun. 2013;434(2):316–21. https://doi.org/10.1016/j.bbrc.2013.03.048.
18. Europa TA, Nel M, Heckmann JM. A review of the histopathological findings in myasthenia gravis: clues to the pathogenesis of treatment-resistance in extraocular muscles. Neuromuscul Disord. 2019;29(5):381–7. https://doi.org/10.1016/j.nmd.2019.03.009.
19. Iqbal S, Ostojic O, Singh K, et al. Expression of mitochondrial fission and fusion regulatory proteins in skeletal muscle during chronic use and disuse. Muscle Nerve. 2013;48(6):963–70. https://doi.org/10.1002/mus.23838.
20. Graham ZA, Harlow L, Bauman WA, et al. Alterations in mitochondrial fission, fusion, and mitophagic protein expression in the gastrocnemius of mice after a sciatic nerve transection. Muscle Nerve. 2018;58(4):592–9. https://doi.org/10.1002/mus.26197.

Diagnostic Criteria for Ocular Myasthenia Gravis

4

4.1 Diagnosis of OMG Based on Clinical Manifestations and Confirmatory Tests

The diagnosis of OMG is mainly based on [1]: (1) Clinical manifestations: the clinical characteristics of fluctuating ocular muscle paralysis; (2) One of the serum AChR-Ab, MuSK-Ab, LRP4-Ab is positive; (3) Positive Edrophonium test or Neostigmine test; (4) Electrophysiological examination: positive repetitive nerve electrical stimulation decay or abnormal single fiber electromyography; (5) Effective treatment with acetylcholinesterase inhibitors. If the first criterion and any one of the other 2–5 are met, and other diseases causing ocular muscle paralysis are excluded, a clear diagnosis can be made.

Suggested diagnostic approach for OMG is as follows (Fig. 4.1):

Q. Zhou, J. Chen, *Ocular Myasthenia Gravis*, Experts' Perspectives on Medical Advances,
https://doi.org/10.1007/978-981-96-1245-1_4

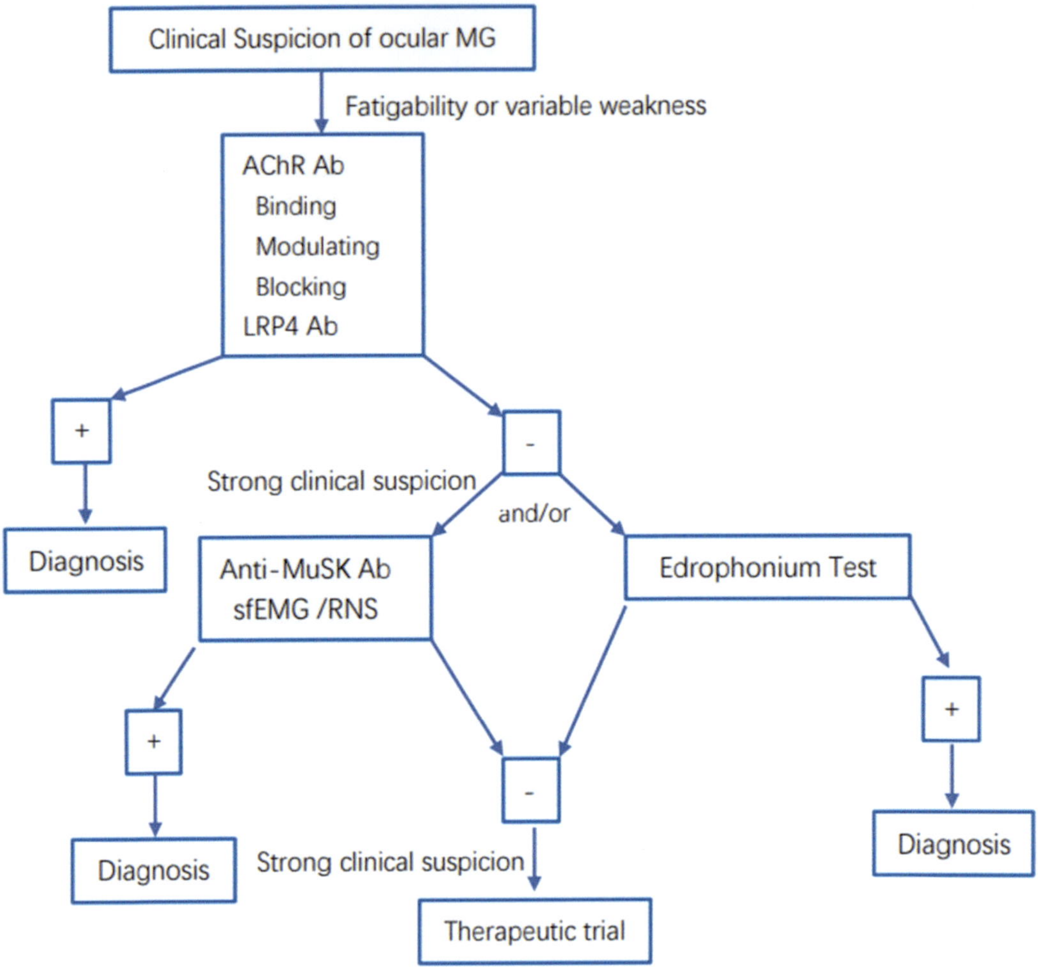

Fig. 4.1 Suggested diagnostic approach for ocular myasthenia gravis (OMG) [1]
Note: *OMG* ocular myasthenia gravis, *AChR-Ab* acetylcholine receptor antibody, *MuSK-Ab* muscle-specific tyrosine kinase receptor antibody, *LRP4-Ab* low-density lipoprotein receptor-related protein 4 antibody, *sfEMG* single fiber electromyography, *RNS* repetitive nerve stimulation test

Reference

1. Fortin E, Cestari DM, Weinberg DH. Ocular myasthenia gravis: an update on diagnosis and treatment. Curr Opin Ophthalmol. 2018;29(6):477–484. https://doi.org/10.1097/ICU.0000000000000526.

5 Clinical Manifestations of Ocular Myasthenia Gravis

5.1 Fluctuating and Fatigable Ptosis and Diplopia in OMG

Ptosis and diplopia are typical manifestations of OMG. These ocular muscles weakness has bilateral asymmetry, fluctuation, and shows the characteristics of being lighter in the morning and heavier in the evening, worsening after activity, and improving after rest or use of acetylcholinesterase inhibitors. The reasons why the NMJ of the extraocular muscles is more susceptible to impact than the NMJ of the skeletal muscles are as follows: (1) fewer synaptic folds, fewer postsynaptic AChR and Na+ channels, and a lower safety factor [1]; (2) susceptible to higher neuronal discharge frequency, prone to fatigue; (3) less expression of intrinsic complement regulatory factors, more susceptible to complement-mediated damage [2].

Ocular muscle weakness can involve a single extraocular muscle or all extraocular muscles [3, 4]. Therefore, OMG can be confused with neurological diseases such as cranial nerve III, IV, or VI or internuclear ophthalmoplegia, an important distinguishing point is that ocular muscle weakness shows fluctuating changes and fatigue. For each patient, a fatigue test should be performed. The diplopia of OMG patients has various forms, such as vertical diplopia and horizontal diplopia. Fluctuating diplopia symptoms can highly suggest OMG. Continuous upward gaze can cause or worsen ptosis or diplopia [5]. Persistent fixation in the direction where diplopia is most pronounced can cause or exacerbate symptoms of diplopia [6]. In cases of mild extraocular muscle paralysis, alternate cover tests or Maddox rod tests can help detect small degrees of strabismus.

Research reports found that diplopia and ptosis occurred separately in 27% and 21% of OMG patients, respectively, and approximately 52% of OMG patients had both ptosis and diplopia [7, 8]. Ptosis can be unilateral or bilateral, usually presenting asymmetry [9]. When the patient maintains a long upward gaze, the symptoms of ptosis become more pronounced [10, 11]. For patients with ptosis, the drooping or more severely drooping side will compensatorily cause an increase in bilateral neural innervation, leading to a pseudoelevation of the bilateral eyelid position, which is due to the bilateral equal innervation of the eyelid (Hering's law) [12]. Although ptosis is the most common symptom in OMG patients, it is not a specific symptom and can also be caused by diseases such as levator aponeurosis tear, Horner's syndrome, oculomotor nerve paralysis, or congenital ptosis [13].

5.2 Cogan's Lid Twitch Sign Is Another Characteristic Manifestation of OMG

Cogan's lid twitch sign is another characteristic manifestation of OMG, which is characterized by a transient widening of the palpebral fissure when looking down to straight ahead. Singman et al.

Q. Zhou, J. Chen, *Ocular Myasthenia Gravis*, Experts' Perspectives on Medical Advances,
https://doi.org/10.1007/978-981-96-1245-1_5

[14] reported its sensitivity to be 75%, with a specificity close to 99%.

5.3 Ocular Myasthenia Gravis Often Presents with Bilateral Orbicularis Oculi Weakness

Bilateral orbicularis oculi muscle weakness often occurs in OMG, but not in other causes of extraocular muscle paralysis, so for suspected OMG patients, orbicularis oculi muscle function should be checked. The involvement of the orbicularis oculi muscle is manifested as a widening of the palpebral fissure after lightly closing the eyes, presenting a "squinting" state, known as the "peek sign."

When a patient is suspected of having OMG based on history and clinical presentation, the same diagnostic tests as for generalized myasthenia gravis (GMG) should be performed to confirm the diagnosis, such as the tensilon test, neostigmine test, ice pack test or rest test, antibody detection, and neurophysiological tests. The condition of the facial, pharyngeal, respiratory, or limb muscles should be carefully examined, as involvement of these muscles suggests GMG.

References

1. Khanna S, Porter J. Conservation of synapse-signaling pathways at the extraocular muscle neuromuscular junction. Ann N Y Acad Sci. 2002;956:394–6.
2. Kaminski H, Li Z, Richmonds C, et al. Complement regulators in extraocular muscle and experimental autoimmune myasthenia gravis. Exp Neurol. 2004;189(2):333–42. https://doi.org/10.1016/j.expneurol.2004.06.005.
3. Evoli A, Tonali P, Bartoccioni E, et al. Ocular myasthenia: diagnostic and therapeutic problems. Acta Neurol Scand. 1988;77(1):31–5. https://doi.org/10.1111/j.1600-0404.1988.tb06970.x.
4. Mansukhani SA, Bothun ED, Diehl NN, et al. Incidence and ocular features of pediatric myasthenias. Am J Ophthalmol. 2019;200:242–9. https://doi.org/10.1016/j.ajo.2019.01.004.
5. Kee HJ, Yang HK, Hwang JM, et al. Evaluation and validation of sustained upgaze combined with the ice-pack test for ocular myasthenia gravis in Asians. Neuromuscul Disord. 2019;29(4):296–301. https://doi.org/10.1016/j.nmd.2018.12.011.
6. Osher RH, Glaser JS. Myasthenic sustained gaze fatigue. Am J Ophthalmol. 1980;89(3):443–5. https://doi.org/10.1016/0002-9394(80)90018-5.
7. Hong Y, Kwon S, Kim B, et al. Prognosis of ocular myasthenia in Korea: a retrospective multicenter analysis of 202 patients. J Neurol Sci. 2008;273(1-2):10–4.
8. Binks S, Vincent A, Palace J. Myasthenia gravis: a clinical-immunological update. J Neurol. 2016;263(4):826–34. https://doi.org/10.1007/s00415-015-7963-5.
9. Evoli A, Alboini P, Damato V, et al. Myasthenia gravis with antibodies to MuSK: an update. Ann N Y Acad Sci. 2018;1412(1):82–9. https://doi.org/10.1111/nyas.13518.
10. Bucy Paul C. Walsh and hoyt's clinical neuro-ophthalmology, 4th edition, volume 2: edited and revised by Neil R. Miller. Br J Ophthalmol. 1985;24(4)
11. Zouvelou V, Papathanasiou A, Koros C, et al. Pure ocular anti-musk myasthenia under no immunosuppressive treatment. Muscle Nerve. 2013;48(3):464. https://doi.org/10.1002/mus.23847.
12. Gay A, ML S, Windsor C. Hering's law, the levators, and their relationship in disease states. Arch Ophthalmol. 1967;77:157–60.
13. Rajasekharan C, Anishkumar V, Suresh M. Ice pack test: is it obsolete? BMJ Case Rep. 2011:bcr0420114066. https://doi.org/10.1136/bcr.04.2011.4066.
14. Singman E, Matta N, Silbert D. Use of the Cogan lid twitch to identify myasthenia gravis. J Neuroophthalmol. 2011;31(3):239–40. https://doi.org/10.1097/WNO.0b013e3182224b92.

6 Clinical Examination Methods for Ocular Myasthenia Gravis

Non-drug tests not only help to improve the diagnosis rate of OMG, but are also simple and easy to perform, mainly including the ice pack test, fatigue test, rest and sleep test, forced eye closure test, neostigmine test, or tensilon test.

6.1 The Ice Pack Test Is a Simple, Safe, Effective, Quick, and Repeatable Clinical Method to Assist in the Diagnosis of OMG

The Ice Pack Test is a simple, safe, effective, quick, and repeatable clinical method for assisting in the diagnosis of OMG. Its principle is mainly that the low temperature state can inhibit the activity of acetylcholinesterase, thereby increasing the utilization rate of neurotransmitters and improving synaptic transmission. This test has high sensitivity (94%) and strong specificity (97%) [1]. Only a few patients with myasthenic ptosis do not respond to the Ice Pack Test [2]. Placing an ice pack on the eyelid for 2~5 min, if the width of the palpebral fissure increases by ≥2 mm (as shown in Fig. 6.1a and b) or the degree of strabismus improves by more than half, it is considered a positive Ice Pack Test. For patients with mild ptosis of OMG, it is advisable to ask the patient to keep looking up for 5 min to cause eyelid fatigue before performing the Ice Pack Test or repeating the Ice Pack Test has a better effect [3]. Patients should stop using acetylcholinesterase inhibitors 4~6 h before the Ice Pack Test. Studies have shown that the Ice Pack Test improves ptosis more significantly than the rest test alone [4, 5], possibly because the eyelid gets rest during the ice pack application [6]. Therefore, when performing the Ice Pack Test clinically, decide whether to perform the fatigue post-Ice Pack Test and repeat the Ice Pack Test based on the patient's response. The mechanism of this test is not fully understood, and current research believes that low temperature can improve synaptic transmission at the end plate [7], enhance muscle excitation-contraction coupling [1], inhibit acetylcholinesterase activity, increase the availability of neurotransmitters, improve synaptic transmission, and thus improve the symptoms of ptosis and diplopia [3].

Q. Zhou, J. Chen, *Ocular Myasthenia Gravis*, Experts' Perspectives on Medical Advances,
https://doi.org/10.1007/978-981-96-1245-1_6

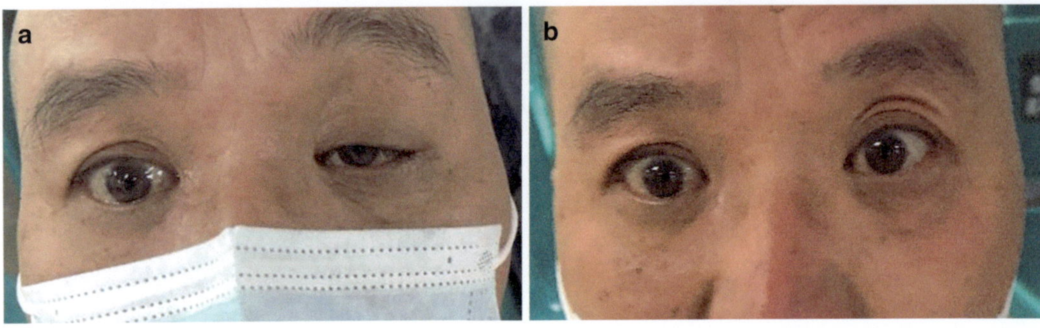

Fig. 6.1 Changes in palpebral fissure height before and after the Ice Pack Test for left eye ptosis. (**a**) Before the Ice Pack Test, the left eye has ptosis, with a palpebral fissure height of 4 mm. (**b**) After the Ice Pack Test, the ptosis of the left eye is significantly improved, with a palpebral fissure height of 11 mm

6.2 Fatigue Test

The Fatigue Test is when the patient continuously looks up with their eyes open, and then the eyelid and extraocular muscles cause ptosis or diplopia to gradually worsen due to fatigue, which is considered a positive Fatigue Test [3]. The sensitivity and specificity of the Fatigue Test for diagnosing OMG are 45.6% and 87.5%, respectively [3].

6.3 Rest and Sleep Tests have High Sensitivity and Specificity

The principle of the rest and sleep test is based on the characteristic improvement of muscle weakness symptoms in patients with OMG after rest. After the patient rests with their eyes closed in a quiet, dark room for 30 min, symptoms such as drooping eyelids and double vision are significantly relieved compared to before rest, but symptoms and signs of OMG reappear within 30 s~5 min, which is a positive result. Rest and sleep tests have high sensitivity and specificity, which are 99% and 91%, respectively [8].

6.4 The Forced Eye Closure Test Is a Simple, Quick, Noninvasive, and Valuable Clinical Screening Test to Assist in the Diagnosis of OMG

The forced eyelid closure test (FECT) is a simple, quick, noninvasive, and valuable clinical screening test developed from the Cogan lid twitch (CLT) to assist in the diagnosis of OMG. The patient is instructed to close their eyelids tightly for 5~10 s, then quickly open their eyes and stare at a target. The observer sits in front of the patient at a distance of 0.6 m~1 m, at the same height as the patient's eyes, and uses their finger to press and fix the eyebrows to minimize the action of the frontal muscle. If the eyelid excessively contracts upwards and then droops, it is a positive result. When the eyes are closed, the orbicularis oculi (OO) muscle contracts tightly, while the levator palpebrae superioris (LPS) is completely relaxed; when the eyelids are immediately opened, the balance between the LPS and its antagonist OO changes. At this time, the contraction force of the LPS is greater than the already fatigued OO, and the eyelid appears to be transiently raised excessively, which is temporary, because the eyelid droops again as the LPS becomes fatigued. Studies have shown that FECT has a high sensitivity (94%) and specificity (91.7%~100%) for the diagnosis of OMG, which is not inferior to CLT in terms of sensitivity and specificity, but false positives occur in Lambert-Eaton myasthenic syndrome (LEMS) and decompensated urethritis [9].

6.5 Tensilon Test or Neostigmine Test

Tensilon, also known as edrophonium chloride, is a short-acting and reversible acetylcholinesterase inhibitor. The principle is to inhibit the breakdown of acetylcholine, thereby increasing its concentration at the neuromuscular junction. As the neurotransmitter at the neuromuscular junction increases, it binds to the postsynaptic receptor, causing changes in the ion channel, generating action potentials, and thus causing muscle contraction [10]. The sensitivity of the tensilon test in diagnosing OMG and GMG is 86% and 95%, respectively [11]. The initial dose for intravenous injection is 2 mg, which starts to take effect after 10~30 s. If it does not take effect after 45~60 s, an additional 2~4 mg is added, up to a maximum of 10 mg [12]. Once a positive result is obtained, no further injection is needed. Common side effects of this test include excessive salivation, sweating, nausea, and muscle tremors, etc. There are also rare serious adverse reactions such as hypotension and bradycardia, with an incidence rate of 0.16% [13]. It is best to give the patient an intravenous injection of 0.4 Atropine is used to prevent severe adverse reactions, and if they occur, 0.5 mg of atropine should be immediately injected intravenously. In addition, the tensilon trial has potential cardiovascular adverse reactions, so caution is needed when used in patients with heart disease or those who have used atrioventricular conduction blocking drugs such as digoxin or β-receptor blockers. The tensilon trial may also complicate the condition due to cholinergic side effects [13]. There have been reports of false positive results in motor neuron diseases, LEMS, and central lesions (including brainstem gliomas and pineal germinomas) [14-16].

The neostigmine test (NT) is fast-acting and long-lasting, allowing for a full observation of changes in ptosis, diplopia, and hypophasis and is safer and more reliable. Adults are given a muscular injection of 1.0 mg~1.5 mg of neostigmine and a simultaneous muscular injection of 0.5 mg of atropine to alleviate M-type cholinergic side effects; the pediatric dose is reduced, with a muscular injection of 0.02~0.04 mg/kg of neostigmine, with a maximum dose not exceeding 1.0 mg, and bromopride is discontinued 6~8 h before the test [17]. Before the injection, the most affected muscle group is selected according to the QMG, and a record is made every 10~15 min before and after the injection, for a total of 60 min. The absolute score at the time of the most significant improvement is recorded, and the relative score is calculated to determine the result. The relative score = (pre-test record score − post-injection record score)/pre-test record score × 100%, a relative score value <25% is negative, 25%~60% is suspiciously positive, >60% is positive [18]. If the test result is negative, the diagnosis of OMG cannot be ruled out [17].

6.6 Method of Strabismus Degree Examination for OMG Patients with Diplopia—Red Filter Plus Prism Method

The operation method for examining the degree of strabismus in patients with diplopia is as follows (as shown in Fig. 6.2): Red filter plus prism method, the patient is instructed to place the prism and red glass separately on both eyes, look at the flashlight at 33 cm, ask the patient about the diplopia distance, start with a small degree prism, gradually increase the prism degree, until the patient can only see one light from seeing one red light and one white light, then the degree of this prism is the strabismus degree of this gaze eye. Due to the subjective factors of both the examiner and the examinee during the measurement process, to ensure the accuracy of the data, each patient should be measured at least three times at

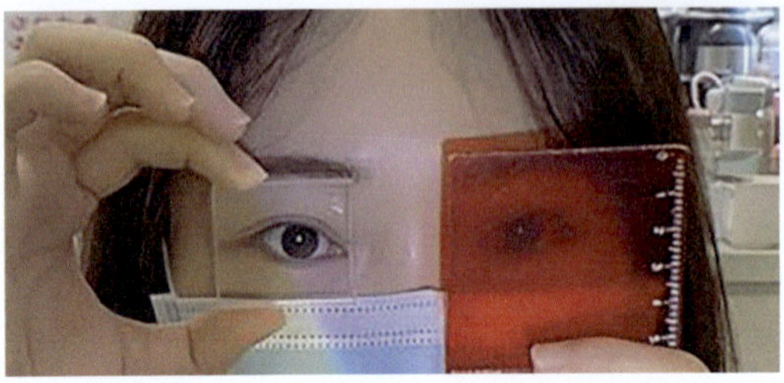

Fig. 6.2 Schematic representation of the red filter combined with the prism method
The patient is instructed to place the prism and red glass separately on both eyes, look at the flashlight

different times, and the average value is taken as the final value. The same method is used to check the strabismus degree of both eyes at 5 m.

References

1. Yamamoto D, Imai T, Tsuda E, et al. Effect of local cooling on excitation-contraction coupling in myasthenic muscle: another mechanism of ice-pack test in myasthenia gravis. Clin Neurophysiol. 2017;128(11):2309–17. https://doi.org/10.1016/j.clinph.2017.08.030.
2. Golnik K, Pena R, Lee A, et al. An ice test for the diagnosis of myasthenia gravis. Ophthalmology. 1999;106(7):1282–6. https://doi.org/10.1016/s0161-6420(99)00709-5.
3. Gay A, ML S, Windsor C. Hering's law, the levators, and their relationship in disease states. Arch Ophthalmol. 1967;77:157–60.
4. Marinos E, Buzzard K, Fraser C, et al. Evaluating the temperature effects of ice and heat tests on ptosis due to myasthenia gravis. Eye (Lond). 2018;32(8):1387–91. https://doi.org/10.1038/s41433-018-0101-8.
5. Kubis K, Danesh-Meyer H, Savino P, et al. The ice test versus the rest test in myasthenia gravis. Ophthalmology. 2000;107:1995–8.
6. Movaghar M, Slavin M. Effect of local heat versus ice on blepharoptosis resulting from ocular myasthenia. Ophthalmology. 2000;107:2209–14.
7. Borenstein S, Desmedt J. Local cooling in myasthenia. Improvement of neuromuscular failure. Arch Neurol. 1975;32:152–7.
8. Odel J, Winterkorn J, Behrens M. The sleep test for myasthenia gravis. A safe alternative to Tensilon. J Clin Neuroophthalmol. 1991;11(4):288–92.
9. Apinyawasisuk S, Zhou X, Tian J, et al. Validity of forced eyelid closure test: a novel clinical screening test for ocular myasthenia gravis. J Neuroophthalmol. 2017;37(3):253–7. https://doi.org/10.1097/WNO.0000000000000514.
10. Pasnoor M, Dimachkie M, Farmakidis C, et al. Diagnosis of myasthenia gravis. Neurol Clin. 2018;36(2):261–74. https://doi.org/10.1016/j.ncl.2018.01.010.
11. Okun M, Charriez C, Bhatti M, et al. Tensilon and the diagnosis of myasthenia gravis: are we using the tensilon test too much? Neurologist. 2001;7(5):295–9.
12. Al-Haidar M, Benatar M, Kaminski H. Ocular myasthenia. Neurol Clin. 2018;36(2):241–51. https://doi.org/10.1016/j.ncl.2018.01.003.
13. Ing EB, Ing SY, Ing T, et al. The complication rate of edrophonium testing for suspected myasthenia gravis. Can J Ophthalmol. 2000;35(3):141–5. https://doi.org/10.1016/s0008-4182(00)80007-1.
14. Seybold ME. The office Tensilon test for ocular myasthenia gravis. Arch Neurol. 1986;43(08):842–3.
15. Dirr LY, Donofrio PD, Patton JF, Troost BT, et al. A false-positive edrophonium test in a patient with a brainstem glioma. Neurology. 1989;39(06):865–7.
16. Fierro BCG, Filosto L, Carbone N, Lupo I. Ocular pseudomyasthenia: report of a case with a pineal region tumor. J Neurol Sci. 1991;12(06):593–6.
17. 常婷. 中国重症肌无力诊断和治疗指南(2020版)[J].中国神经免疫学和神经病学杂志, 2021;28(01):1–12.
18. Dantao P, Xianhao X, Ziyu S. Research on the improved result judgment method of Neostigmine test. Chinese J Neuroimmunol Neurol. 2007;01:1–3.

Serological Test for Ocular Myasthenia Gravis

7

The pathogenesis of OMG is closely related to antibody mediation, and the detection of serum antibodies is an important means of diagnosing OMG. Relevant antibodies include: acetylcholine receptor antibody (AChR-Ab), muscle-specific tyrosine kinase antibody (MuSK-Ab), and low-density lipoprotein receptor-related protein 4 antibody (LRP4-Ab), etc. OMG with both AChR-Ab and MuSK-Ab negative is called double seronegative OMG (dSN-OMG).

7.1 Acetylcholine Receptor Antibody Has the Highest Specificity for Ocular Myasthenia Gravis

In 1973, Patrick and Lindstrom first reported AChR-Ab [1], AChR-Ab positivity is the most specific serological test for diagnosing OMG, with a specificity of about 98~100% in patients with suggestive symptoms and signs [2]. This antibody test has become the most specific diagnostic aid for OMG, especially in thymoma patients or family members, false positives are rare [3, 4]. AChR-Ab primarily consists of IgG1 and IgG3 subclasses [5], both have complement activity, can activate the complement on the postsynaptic membrane, leading to the loss of AChR and destruction of its characteristic structure, which is necessary for effective signal transduction [6]. In addition, because AChR-Ab is bivalent, it can cause AChR endocytosis and destruction (antigen regulation) after cross-linking with AChR [7]. Autoantibodies binding around the receptor binding site can directly interfere with the activation of AChR by acetylcholine [8]. AChR-Ab subtypes include binding, modulating, and blocking [9, 10]. Binding AChR-Ab is the most important one, modulating AChR-Ab can increase detection sensitivity, blocking AChR-Ab has lower clinical utility because it cannot be detected alone [9, 10].

Methods for detecting AChR-Ab mainly include radioimmunoassay and enzyme-linked immunosorbent assay (ELISA). The minimum titer of ELISA detection is the same as that of radioimmunoassay, but the specificity and sensitivity of radioimmunoassay are higher than ELISA [2444, 245], with a specificity close to 100% [11]. Therefore, when the radioimmunoassay is positive, it can be diagnosed as MG with the clinical manifestations of fluctuating myasthenia. In addition, cell-based assay (CBA) is often used for patients with both AChR-Ab and MuSK-Ab negative. For those AChR-Ab positive MG patients, the detection of acetylcholine receptor by CBA usually indicates only clinically mild and good prognosis MG patients [12], due to the lack of commercial production and complex operation process, it is not yet used as a routine detection method.

Studies have reported that the positive rates of AChR-Ab in GMG and OMG patients are

Q. Zhou, J. Chen, *Ocular Myasthenia Gravis*, Experts' Perspectives on Medical Advances,
https://doi.org/10.1007/978-981-96-1245-1_7

80%~90% and 50%~60%, respectively [13]. Evoli et al. [14] reported a study of 48 OMG patients that only 45.5% of patients tested positive for AChR-Ab. AChR-Ab positivity has a high predictive value for the diagnosis of MG; however, the negative predictive value is relatively low, especially for OMG. More than half of OMG patients have a negative AChR-Ab, so a negative AChR-Ab test cannot rule out OMG [2]. The level of AChR-Ab is not significantly related to the severity or progression of the disease [11, 13], thus high antibody levels are not sufficient to predict the severity of symptoms and prognosis, and are therefore not usually used to guide treatment decision-making.

7.2 The Positive Rate of Muscle-Specific Tyrosine Kinase Receptor Antibody in OMG Patients Is Low

In 2001, Hoch et al. first reported the presence of MuSK-Ab in MG patients [15]. MuSK is a transmembrane tyrosine kinase receptor, a signaling molecule that plays a key role in the formation of mature and functional neuromuscular junctions. The activation of MuSK requires complex interactions between its co-receptor LRP4, Agrin, and the intracellular adapter protein Dok-7. MuSK activation downstream signaling can induce pre- and postsynaptic differentiation, the most important of which is causing AChR to cluster in the postsynaptic membrane; therefore, MuSK signaling defects are an important cause of MG [16]. In addition to blocking neuromuscular transmission, MuSK antibodies also downregulate important postsynaptic genes and proteins at the neuromuscular junction, induce cell cycle arrest and inhibit cell proliferation, disrupt muscle regeneration mechanisms, and cause progressive muscle atrophy [17]. Unlike AChR-Ab, and do not activate complement [18]. In vitro studies have shown that IgG4 antibodies to MuSK block the interaction between MuSK and LRP4, thereby preventing the clustering of AChR, which also explains the neuromuscular junction transmission disorder in OMG.

For AChR-Ab negative MG patients, radioimmunoassay or ELISA should be used to detect IgG4 antibodies to MuSk. MuSK-Ab positive MG is usually more likely to involve the bulbar region than AChR-Ab positive MG, and other phenotypes including OMG may also occur [19]. The radioimmunoassay is highly sensitive and can detect low concentrations of antibodies, although some MuSK-Ab are conformation-dependent, so this method does not bind to the extracellular domain of soluble MuSK-Ab [20]. Cell-based detection methods have certain advantages in detecting this conformation-dependent MuSK-Ab, but it is difficult to maintain the same specificity as the radioimmunoassay [20]. Selective detection of IgG antibodies to MuSK-Ab (excluding IgM antibodies) can increase the specificity of cell-based detection methods [21].

In all MG patients, about 6% tested positive for MuSK-Ab [22, 23], and in AChR-Ab negative MG patients, about 40% tested positive for MuSK-Ab [22]. The reason for the lower incidence of MuSK-Ab positive MG patients in Northern Europe and higher incidence in the Mediterranean may be due to geographical and genetic differences [11, 24]. In the Japanese population, MuSK-Ab MG patients are uncommon, with a total incidence rate of 2~3% [25, 26]. Until now, the detection of MuSK-Ab in AChR-Ab positive patients is still very rare [27]. The detection rate of MuSK-Ab in OMG is low, and MuSK-Ab should still be tested in the case of serum negativity for AChR-Ab and LRP4-Ab. Evoli et al. [19] found in a retrospective study that out of 82 MuSK-Ab positive patients, only 3 patients presented with pure ocular involvement, indicating that MuSK-Ab positive patients rarely present with only ocular symptoms, often accompanied by severe clinical symptoms. Studies have shown that the incidence of MuSK-Ab positive OMG progressing to GMG is high [28, 29]. The titer of MuSK antibodies seems to be related to the severity of the disease [30, 31]. The rate of complete stable remission in MuSK-Ab positive patients is lower than in AChR-Ab positive MG patients [19].

MuSK-Ab positive patients are usually unrelated to thymic abnormalities. A recent retrospective multicenter study found that good clinical remission was not achieved after thymectomy [32]. On the other hand, in patients with MUSK-Ab positivity detected by CBA, 23% of patients were found to have thyroid hyperplasia [20].

7.3 The Positive Rate of Low-Density Lipoprotein Receptor-Related Protein 4 Antibody in OMG Patients Is High

LRP4-Ab is a new pathogenic antibody found in MG in recent years. It is a single subunit transmembrane protein and belongs to the low-density lipoprotein receptor family. In the neuromuscular junction, LRP4 acts as a receptor for Agrin, and LRP4-Ab can disrupt the interaction between LRP4 and Agrin, thereby disrupting the function of the neuromuscular junction by inhibiting Agrin-induced MuSK activation and AChR aggregation [33, 34]. The main types of LRP4-Ab are lgG1 and lgG2 subclasses, similar to AChR, they produce pathogenic effects by activating the complement [35]. Studies have shown that cell-based detection methods are usually used to detect LRP4-Ab [35], and ELISA are occasionally used for detection [36]. So far, there is no evidence that MG can be induced by passively transferring human LRP4-Ab into animals. The pathogenicity of LRP4-Ab in OMG is not yet fully determined.

Because of the different methods used to detect antibodies and the different populations tested, there is a large variation in the detection rate of LRP4-Ab in MG patients [35]. In this largest study with samples from 10 different countries, 19% of seronegative (both AChR-Ab and MuSK-Ab negative) MG patients were found to have LRP4-Ab, and 27% of seronegative OMG patients were tested for LRP4-Ab [35]. In addition, this study detected LRP4-Ab in 8% of AChR-Ab positive patients, 15% of MuSK-Ab positive patients, and 4% of other neuroimmune disease patients [35]. No cases of thymoma were found in LRP4-Ab positive MG patients, suggesting that thymoma may not be common in this subtype of MG [35]. 34% of LRP4-Ab positive MG patients achieved relief (completely stable or drug-stable) after using pyridostigmine bromide, and about 70% of LRP4-Ab positive MG patients needed combined immunosuppressive treatment to achieve satisfactory results. LRP4-Ab is not a specific antibody for MG and can also be detected in 23% of motor neuron diseases [35, 37] as well as in myasthenia gravis and optic neuritis patients [35]. The IgG1 subtype is the main antibody type in MG patients and patients with amyotrophic lateral sclerosis and can bind with complement [35]. MG antibody testing usually does not include LRP-4 antibody, so sending this separate test may be useful in seronegative OMG patients.

Chinese scholar Li et al. [38] collected serum samples from 2172 MG patients in most regions of our country and found 16 (0.8%) LRP4-MG patients, among which there were three AChR-Ab and LRP4-Ab positive MG patients; 13 (2.9%) LRP4-MG patients were found among 455 seronegative MG patients, the male to female ratio among these 13 patients was 1:1.6, with children accounting for 53.8%; as many as 91.7% of cases clinically involved ocular muscles, and 58.3% of cases were purely ocular muscle involvement. These research results found that the majority of LRP4-Ab positive MG patients start with ocular myasthenia, and the incidence of purely involving the eyes is higher, indicating that LRP4-Ab plays an important role in the occurrence and development of OMG, so for seronegative antibody and clinically suspected OMG patients, LRP4-Ab should be screened. Compared with AChR-Ab or MuSK-Ab positive patients, LRP4-Ab positive patients have a lighter course of disease, such as LRP4-Ab patients without myasthenic crisis [39, 40].

7.4 Striated Muscle Antibody Expected to Become a Predictive Marker for Thymoma in Patients with Myasthenia Gravis

Various striated muscle antibodies can be detected in MG patients, mainly including Titin antibodies, RyR antibodies, Kv1.4 antibodies, etc. Anti-striated body antibodies can be detected in MG patients with thymoma and late-onset MG patients, so they are expected to be a predictive marker for thymoma in MG patients.

7.4.1 Titin Antibody

In 1990, the autoantibody of the giant myofibrillar protein Titin (up to 4200 kDa) was first detected in patients with severe myasthenia gravis (MG) [41]. Titin is not only the largest known filamentous intracellular protein, but also the third most abundant striated muscle protein, and a major component of muscle cell actin, including skeletal muscle and myocardium [42, 43]. Titin plays a crucial role in the development, elasticity, and signal transmission of sarcomeres, as well as the stability of muscle fibers. If Titin is damaged, it will affect muscle contraction [43, 44].

In AChR-Ab positive MG patients, Titin antibody positivity accounts for 20~40%, and is significantly related to age, as low as 6% in early-onset OMG patients, and as high as 50-80% in late-onset OMG patients [45]. Studies have shown that Titin and RyR epitopes are expressed on the tumor epithelial cells of cortical thymoma [46]. The sensitivity of Titin antibody in diagnosing thymoma is 82.1%, and the specificity is 52.5% [47]. In MG patients with concurrent thymoma, the positivity rate of Titin antibody is as high as 70%~90% [18]. The presence of Titin antibodies often indicates severe MG with thymoma and mild myopathy. The positivity rate of Titin antibodies in AChR-Ab negative OMG patients is about 33%, suggesting that Titin antibody positivity is helpful in the diagnosis of AChR-Ab negative OMG patients [48].

7.4.2 RyR Antibody

RyR is a calcium channel in the sarcoplasmic reticulum, which opens during muscle membrane depolarization and participates in muscle contraction by releasing calcium from the muscle membrane into the cytoplasm. The RyR subtype plays an important role in skeletal muscle excitation-contraction coupling, and if damaged, it can lead to muscle weakness [49]. Studies have reported that RyR antibodies are significantly associated with thymoma, and RyR antibodies are detected in 70% of thymoma MG and 14% of late-onset MG [50, 51]. RyR antibodies are significantly associated with thymoma, indicating severe MG [50, 51].

7.4.3 Kv1.4 Antibody

Kv1.4 is a voltage-gated potassium channel, concentrated on the axonal membrane, and also found in the endocardium [52]. Kv1.4 antibodies may cross-react with the voltage-gated potassium channels of the myocardial membrane in MG patients. Research results found that Kv1.4 antibodies were detected in 50% of MG patients with concurrent myocarditis, and 28% of other MG patients, especially in late-onset and thymoma-related MG patients [53]. Kv1.4 antibodies are common in Japanese GMG patients, indicating a more severe condition, prone to crisis, and poor prognosis [43, 44]. Kv1.4 antibodies have also been found in Caucasians, indicating mild symptoms or mainly presenting as OMG [54].

7.5 Other Antibodies

In recent years, Agrin antibodies and cortactin antibodies have also been found in the serum of MG patients. Studies have shown that the incidence of these antibodies in seronegative MG is higher than in seropositive MG, providing a direction for the exploration of seronegative MG [55, 56].

7.5.1 Agrin Antibody

Agrin is a neurogenic polysaccharide secreted by the terminals of motor neurons, which can promote the aggregation of AChR on the postsynaptic membrane; muscle cells also express Agrin, but only motor neurons can produce a selectively spliced subtype called "z-agrin," which can activate the complex composed of LRP4, MuSK, and AChR. This complex regulates the formation, maintenance, and regeneration of neuromuscular junctions [33, 57-59]. Without Agrin or only with z-agrin, the postsynaptic membrane of the neuromuscular junction cannot differentiate normally, and animals will die shortly after birth [60, 61]. Therefore, Agrin antibodies also play an important pathogenic role in MG. Agrin antibodies appear in 4% of MG patients, more common in early-onset female MG patients, with clinical symptoms varying from mild to severe, and treatment responses vary [48].

7.5.2 Cortactin Antibody

In skeletal muscle, cortactin binds to actin, promotes actin assembly, interacts with the Agrin-LRP4-MuSK complex, and promotes the regulation of actin aggregation and AChR aggregation at the postsynaptic membrane of the neuromuscular junction [14, 62]. Approximately 20% of seronegative MG patients tested positive for cortactin antibodies, while only 4.8% of AChR-Ab positive MG patients tested positive for cortactin antibodies [63]. However, cortactin antibodies can also be detected in up to 5% of healthy controls and 10%~15% of patients with other autoimmune diseases [63, 64], and cortactin antibodies can also be detected in 20% of patients with polymyositis [65], the low specificity of cortactin antibodies makes it insufficient as a biomarker for diagnosing MG.

References

1. Patrick J, Lindstrom J. Autoimmune response to acetylcholine receptor. Science. 1973;180(4088):871–2. https://doi.org/10.1126/science.180.4088.871.
2. Benatar M. A systematic review of diagnostic studies in myasthenia gravis. Neuromuscul Disord. 2006;16(7):459–67. https://doi.org/10.1016/j.nmd.2006.05.006.
3. Vincent A, Newsom-Davis J. Acetylcholine receptor antibody as a diagnostic test for myasthenia gravis: results in 153 validated cases and 2967 diagnostic assays. Neurol Neurosurg Psychiatry. 1985;48(12):1246–52.
4. Jacobson D. Acetylcholine receptor antibodies in patients with graves' ophthalmopathy. J Neuroophthalmol. 1995;15(3):166–70.
5. Lefvert AK, Cuénoud S, Fulpius BW. Binding properties and subclass distribution of anti-acetylcholine receptor antibodies in myasthenia gravis. J Neuroimmunol. 1981;1(1):125–35. https://doi.org/10.1016/0165-5728(81)90015-1.
6. Engel AG, Arahata K. The membrane attack complex of complement at the endplate in myasthenia gravis. Ann N Y Acad Sci. 1987;505:326–32. https://doi.org/10.1111/j.1749-6632.1987.tb51301.x.
7. Drachman DB, Angus CW, Adams RN, et al. Myasthenic antibodies cross-link acetylcholine receptors to accelerate degradation. N Engl J Med. 1978;298(20):1116–22. https://doi.org/10.1056/nejm197805182982004.
8. Drachman DB, Adams RN, Josifek LF, et al. Functional activities of autoantibodies to acetylcholine receptors and the clinical severity of myasthenia gravis. N Engl J Med. 1982;307(13):769–75. https://doi.org/10.1056/nejm198209233071301.
9. FM H Jr, Lennon VA, Finley J, et al. Clinical correlations of antibodies that bind, block, or modulate human acetylcholine receptors in myasthenia gravis. Ann N Y Acad Sci. 1987;505:526–38. https://doi.org/10.1111/j.1749-6632.1987.tb51321.x.
10. Vincent A, McConville J, Farrugia ME, et al. Seronegative myasthenia gravis. Semin Neurol. 2004;24(1):125–33. https://doi.org/10.1055/s-2004-829589.
11. Gilhus NE, Verschuuren JJ. Myasthenia gravis: subgroup classification and therapeutic strategies. Lancet Neurol. 2015;14(10):1023–36. https://doi.org/10.1016/s1474-4422(15)00145-3.
12. Berrih-Aknin S, Frenkian-Cuvelier M, Eymard B. Diagnostic and clinical classification of autoimmune myasthenia gravis. J Autoimmun. 2014;48(49):143–8. https://doi.org/10.1016/j.jaut.2014.01.003.
13. Roses A, Olanow W, McAdams M. No direct correlation between serum antiacetylcholine receptor antibody levels and clinical state of individual patients with myasthenia gravis. Neurology. 1981;31(2):220–4.
14. Madhavan R, Gong ZL, Ma JJ, et al. The function of cortactin in the clustering of acetylcholine receptors at the vertebrate neuromuscular junction. PLoS One. 2009;4(12):e8478. https://doi.org/10.1371/journal.pone.0008478.
15. Hoch W, McConville J, Helms S, et al. Auto-antibodies to the receptor tyrosine kinase MuSK in patients with myasthenia gravis without acetylcholine receptor antibodies. Nat Med. 2001;7(3):365–8. https://doi.org/10.1038/85520.
16. DeChiara TM, Bowen DC, et al. The receptor tyrosine kinase MuSK is required for neuromuscular junction formation in vivo. Cell. 1996;85:501–12.
17. Boneva N, Frenkian-Cuvelier M, Bidault J, et al. Major pathogenic effects of anti-MuSK anti-

bodies in myasthenia gravis. J Neuroimmunol. 2006;177(1-2):119–31. https://doi.org/10.1016/j.jneuroim.2006.05.017.
18. McConville J, Farrugia M, Beeson D, et al. Detection and characterization of MuSK antibodies in seronegative myasthenia gravis. Ann Neurol. 2004;55(4):580–4. https://doi.org/10.1002/ana.20061.
19. Evoli A, Alboini P, Damato V, et al. Myasthenia gravis with antibodies to MuSK: an update. Ann N Y Acad Sci. 2018;1412(1):82–9. https://doi.org/10.1111/nyas.13518.
20. Tsonis AI, Zisimopoulou P, Lazaridis K, et al. MuSK autoantibodies in myasthenia gravis detected by cell based assay—a multinational study. J Neuroimmunol. 2015;284:10–7. https://doi.org/10.1016/j.jneuroim.2015.04.015.
21. Huda S, Waters P, Woodhall M, et al. IgG-specific cell-based assay detects potentially pathogenic MuSK-Abs in seronegative MG. Neurol Neuroimmunol Neuroinflamm. 2017;4(4):e357. https://doi.org/10.1212/nxi.0000000000000357.
22. Guptill JT, Sanders DB, Evoli A. Anti-musk antibody myasthenia gravis: clinical findings and response to treatment in two large cohorts. Muscle Nerve. 2011;44(1):36–40. https://doi.org/10.1002/mus.22006.
23. Stergiou C, Lazaridis K, Zouvelou V, et al. Titin antibodies in "seronegative" myasthenia gravis—a new role for an old antigen. J Neuroimmunol. 2016;292:108–15. https://doi.org/10.1016/j.jneuroim.2016.01.018.
24. Binks S, Vincent A, Palace J. Myasthenia gravis: a clinical-immunological update. J Neurol. 2016;263(4):826–34. https://doi.org/10.1007/s00415-015-7963-5.
25. Suzuki S, Utsugisawa K, Nagane Y, et al. Clinical and immunological differences between early and late-onset myasthenia gravis in Japan. J Neuroimmunol. 2011;230(1-2):148–52. https://doi.org/10.1016/j.jneuroim.2010.10.023.
26. Zouvelou V, Papathanasiou A, Koros C, et al. Pure ocular anti-musk myasthenia under no immunosuppressive treatment. Muscle Nerve. 2013;48(3):464. https://doi.org/10.1002/mus.23847.
27. Ohta K, Shigemoto K, Kubo S, et al. MuSK antibodies in AChR Ab-seropositive MG vs AChR Ab-seronegative MG. Neurology. 2004;62(11):2132–3. https://doi.org/10.1212/01.wnl.0000129274.12702.92.
28. Galassi G, Mazzoli M, Ariatti A, et al. Antibody profile may predict outcome in ocular myasthenia gravis. Acta Neurol Belg. 2018;118(3):435–43. https://doi.org/10.1007/s13760-018-0943-7.
29. Aguirre F, Villa A. Prognosis of ocular myasthenia gravis in an Argentinian population. Eur Neurol. 2018;79(3-4):113–7. https://doi.org/10.1159/000487132.
30. Bartoccioni E, Scuderi F, Minicuci GM, et al. Anti-MuSK antibodies: correlation with myasthenia gravis severity. Neurology. 2006;67(3):505–7.
31. Niks EH, van Leeuwen Y, Leite MI, et al. Clinical fluctuations in MuSK myasthenia gravis are related to antigen-specific IgG4 instead of IgG1. J Neuroimmunol. 2008;195(1-2):151–6. https://doi.org/10.1016/j.jneuroim.2008.01.013.
32. Kaufman AJ, Palatt J, Sivak M, et al. Thymectomy for myasthenia gravis: complete stable remission and associated prognostic factors in over 1000 cases. Semin Thorac Cardiovasc Surg. 2016;28(2):561–8. https://doi.org/10.1053/j.semtcvs.2016.04.002.
33. Kim N, Stiegler A, Cameron TO, et al. Lrp4 is a receptor for Agrin and forms a complex with MuSK. Cell. 2008;135(2):334–42. https://doi.org/10.1016/j.cell.2008.10.002.
34. Weatherbee S, Anderson KV, Niswander LA. LDL-receptor-related protein 4 is crucial for formation of the neuromuscular junction. Development. 2006;133(24):4993–5000. https://doi.org/10.1242/dev.02696.
35. Zisimopoulou P, Evangelakou P, Tzartos J, et al. A comprehensive analysis of the epidemiology and clinical characteristics of anti-LRP4 in myasthenia gravis. J Autoimmun. 2014;52:139–45. https://doi.org/10.1016/j.jaut.2013.12.004.
36. Zhang B, Tzartos JS, Belimezi M, Ragheb S, Bealmear B, Lewis RA, Xiong WC, Lisak RP, Tzartos SJ, Mei L. Autoantibodies to lipoprotein-related protein 4 in patients with double-seronegative myasthenia gravis. Arch Neurol. 2012;69(4):445–51. https://doi.org/10.1001/archneurol.2011.2393.
37. Rivner MH, Liu S, Quarles B, et al. Agrin and low-density lipoprotein-related receptor protein 4 antibodies in amyotrophic lateral sclerosis patients. Muscle Nerve. 2017;55(3):430–2. https://doi.org/10.1002/mus.25438.
38. Li Y, Zhang Y, Cai G, et al. Anti-LRP4 autoantibodies in Chinese patients with myasthenia gravis. Muscle Nerve. 2017;56(5):938–42. https://doi.org/10.1002/mus.25591.
39. Oh SJ. Muscle-specific receptor tyrosine kinase antibody positive myasthenia gravis current status. J Clin Neurol. 2009;5:53–64.
40. Evoli A, Padua L. Diagnosis and therapy of myasthenia gravis with antibodies to muscle-specific kinase. Autoimmun Rev. 2013;12(9):931–5. https://doi.org/10.1016/j.autrev.2013.03.004.
41. Aarl J, Stefansson K, Marton L, et al. Patients with myasthenia gravis and thymoma have in their sera IgG autoantibodies against titin. J Clin Exp Immunol. 1990;82(2)
42. Bang M, Centner T, Fornoff F, et al. The complete gene sequence of titin, expression of an unusual approximately 700-kDa titin isoform, and its interaction with obscurin identify a novel Z-line to I-band linking system. Circ Res.

2001;89(11):1065–72. https://doi.org/10.1161/hh2301.100981.
43. Linke W, Hamdani N. Gigantic business: titin properties and function through thick and thin. Circ Res. 2014;114(6):1052–68. https://doi.org/10.1161/CIRCRESAHA.114.301286.
44. Linke W. Sense and stretchability: the role of titin and titin-associated proteins in myocardial stress-sensing and mechanical dysfunction. Cardiovasc Res. 2008;77(4):637–48. https://doi.org/10.1016/j.cardiores.2007.03.029.
45. Szczudlik P, Szyluk B, Lipowska M, et al. Antititin antibody in early- and late-onset myasthenia gravis. Acta Neurol Scand. 2014;130(4):229–33. https://doi.org/10.1111/ane.12271.
46. Romi F, Bø L, Skeie GO, Myking A, Aarli JA, Gilhus NE, et al. Titin and ryanodine receptor epitopes are expressed in cortical thymoma along with costimulatory molecules. Neuroimmunology. 2002;128(1-2):82–9.
47. Sommer N, Willcox N, Harcourt G, et al. Myasthenic thymus and thymoma are selectively enriched in acetylcholine receptor-reactive T cells. Ann Neurol. 1990;28(3):312–9.
48. Cordts I, Bodart N, Hartmann K, et al. Screening for lipoprotein receptor-related protein 4-, agrin-, and titin-antibodies and exploring the autoimmune spectrum in myasthenia gravis. J Neurol. 2017;264(6):1193–203. https://doi.org/10.1007/s00415-017-8514-z.
49. Imai T, Tsuda E, Hozuki T, et al. Contribution of anti-ryanodine receptor antibody to impairment of excitation-contraction coupling in myasthenia gravis. Clin Neurophysiol. 2012;123(6):1242–7. https://doi.org/10.1016/j.clinph.2011.10.038.
50. Romi F, Hong Y, Gilhus NE. Pathophysiology and immunological profile of myasthenia gravis and its subgroups. Curr Opin Immunol. 2017;49:9–13. https://doi.org/10.1016/j.coi.2017.07.006.
51. Mygland A, Tysnes OB, Matre R, et al. Ryanodine receptor autoantibodies in myasthenia gravis patients with a thymoma. Ann Neurol. 1992;32(4):589–91. https://doi.org/10.1002/ana.410320419.
52. O'Connell KM, Whitesell JD, Tamkun MM. Localization and mobility of the delayed-rectifer K+ channel Kv2.1 in adult cardiomyocytes. Am J Physiol Heart Circ Physiol. 2008;294(1):H229–37. https://doi.org/10.1152/ajpheart.01038.2007.
53. Kufukihara K, Watanabe Y, Inagaki T, et al. Cytometric cell-based assays for anti-striational antibodies in myasthenia gravis with myositis and/or myocarditis. Sci Rep. 2019;9(1):5284. https://doi.org/10.1038/s41598-019-41730-z.
54. Romi F, Suzuki S, Suzuki N, et al. Anti-voltage-gated potassium channel Kv1.4 antibodies in myasthenia gravis. J Neurol. 2012;259(7):1312–6. https://doi.org/10.1007/s00415-011-6344-y.
55. Yan M, Xing G, Xiong WC, et al. Agrin and LRP4 antibodies as new biomarkers of myasthenia gravis. Ann N Y Acad Sci. 2018;1413(1):126–35. https://doi.org/10.1111/nyas.13573.
56. Cortés-Vicente E, Gallardo E, Martínez MÁ, et al. Clinical characteristics of patients with double-seronegative myasthenia gravis and antibodies to cortactin. JAMA Neurol. 2016;73(9):1099–104. https://doi.org/10.1001/jamaneurol.2016.2032.
57. DeChiara TM, Bowen DC, Valenzuela DM, et al. The receptor tyrosine kinase MuSK is required for neuromuscular junction formation in vivo. Cell. 1996;85:501–12.
58. David JG, David CB, Stitt TN, et al. Clinical characteristics of patients with double-seronegative myasthenia gravis and antibodies to cortactin. Cell. 1996;85:513–23.
59. Zhang B, Luo S, Wang Q, et al. LRP4 serves as a coreceptor of agrin. Neuron. 2008;60(2):285–97. https://doi.org/10.1016/j.neuron.2008.10.006.
60. Gautam M, Noakes P, Moscoso L, et al. Defective neuromuscular synaptogenesis in agrin-deficient mutant mice. Cell. 1996;85:525–35.
61. Burgess RW, Nguyen QT, Son YJ, et al. Alternatively spliced isoforms of nerve- and muscle-derived agrin: their roles at the neuromuscular junction. Neuron. 1999;23:33–44.
62. Peng HB, Xie H, Dai Z. Association of cortactin with developing neuromuscular specializations. Neurocytology. 1997;26:637–50.
63. Illa I, Cortes-Vicente E, Martinez MA, et al. Diagnostic utility of cortactin antibodies in myasthenia gravis. Ann N Y Acad Sci. 2018;1412(1):90–4. https://doi.org/10.1111/nyas.13502.
64. Gallardo E, Martínez-Hernández E, Titulaer MJ, et al. Cortactin autoantibodies in myasthenia gravis. Autoimmun Rev. 2014;13(10):1003–7. https://doi.org/10.1016/j.autrev.2014.08.039.
65. Labrador-Horrillo M, Martínez MA, Selva-O'Callaghan A, et al. Identification of a novel myositis-associated antibody directed against cortactin. Autoimmun Rev. 2014;13(10):1008–12. https://doi.org/10.1016/j.autrev.2014.08.038.

8 Electrophysiological Examination

When the patient's antibody test is negative and OMG needs to be confirmed, neurophysiological testing is particularly important.

8.1 Repetitive Nerve Stimulation Is Most Commonly Used for the Diagnosis of Ocular Myasthenia Gravis

In addition to serological testing, electromyography can be used to support the clinical diagnosis of OMG, especially in seronegative OMG patients. Repetitive nerve stimulation (RNS), as part of electromyographic research, originated at the end of the nineteenth century. After decades of exploration and improvement, it became a routine testing method by the mid-twentieth century and is now the most commonly used neurophysiological examination technique for diagnosing MG.

The frequency of RNS stimulation can be selected, with a lower frequency (2~5 Hz) of repetitive nerve electrical stimulation having a higher positive rate than a high frequency (10~20 Hz) of repetitive nerve electrical stimulation, and causing less pain for the patient. Therefore, MG patients often use low-frequency repetitive nerve electrical stimulation. This technique stimulates the proximal muscle nerves and facial nerves repeatedly, recording the changes in the compound muscle action potential (CMAP) produced by each stimulation. Although RNS will consume acetylcholine vesicles in the presynaptic at this frequency, the amplitude of CMAP in normal neuromuscular junctions can remain stable. For MG patients, repetitive stimulation can cause the endplate potential to drop below the threshold required for each all-or-none muscle fiber action potential; therefore, repetitive stimulation can cause the total amplitude of CMAPs in MG patients to decrease. Usually, the first CMAP is compared with the fourth or fifth CMAP, and a decrease of more than 10% indicates a positive RNS [1]. The sensitivity of RNS in diagnosing OMG is low (11%~35%), but the specificity is high (89%~98%) [2]. RNS can improve its sensitivity by directly detecting the muscles that show weakness clinically, studies have found that testing the orbicularis oculi muscle can help improve the detection rate of OMG [3].

In healthy people, acetylcholine is mobilized from the secondary storage after 1~2 s of repetitive nerve electrical stimulation, which improves the action potential and allows the CMAP to decay stably or slightly improve. In MG, muscle movement causes fatigue, which exacerbates the decline in CMAP amplitude. In other cases, such as Lambert-Eaton myasthenic syndrome, motor neuron disease, and other nerve diseases, a weakened response to slow RNS can be found [4]. Therefore, RNS should be performed simultaneously with routine nerve conduction tests and electromyography to ensure that these other con-

Q. Zhou, J. Chen, *Ocular Myasthenia Gravis*, Experts' Perspectives on Medical Advances,
https://doi.org/10.1007/978-981-96-1245-1_8

ditions are not overlooked. RNS also requires high technical skills, and any movement of the patient, recording electrodes, or nerve stimulators can artificially cause a decrease in RNS response.

8.2 Single Fiber Electromyography Is Superior to Repetitive Nerve Stimulation in the Diagnosis of Ocular Myasthenia Gravis

Single-fiber electromyography (SFEMG) is a highly sensitive detection method in OMG, with higher sensitivity than RNS, but not as specific as RNS [5]. Currently, there are two methods of SFEMG used for diagnosing MG, one is the voluntary contraction method, which requires the subject to actively contract the muscles, measuring the changes in jitter values between muscle fibers innervated by the same motor axon; the other is the passive contraction method, which measures the time changes between nerve stimulation and muscle jitter [6]. This test is usually performed on the orbicularis oculi muscle, frontalis muscle, or interphalangeal joint extensor, and evaluates jitter to understand the contraction state of the muscle. Jitter is defined as the time change to reach the depolarization endplate potential between two muscle fibers innervated by the same nerve branch [7].

Multiple studies have shown that SFEMG is superior to RNS in diagnosing OMG, especially seronegative OMG, with sensitivities of approximately 80% and 94% in OMG and GMG, respectively [8, 9, 10]. The sensitivity and specificity of SFEMG depend on the muscle being studied, with the highest sensitivity for the orbicularis oculi muscle, reaching 94%~99%, and a specificity of 85%~98% [11]. At the same time, studies have found that the initial SFEMG value of the orbicularis oculi muscle has prognostic value in the long-term clinical course of MG patients. A higher average jitter value at the orbicularis oculi muscle may indicate a worsening of the disease in the later stage. Therefore, we chose the orbicularis oculi muscle to evaluate SFEMG [12]. Giannoccaro et al. [13] found that the diagnostic sensitivity and specificity of SFEMG in the orbicularis oculi muscle of OMG patients were 79% and 80%, respectively; they also found that the diagnostic sensitivity is related to clinical manifestations. The sensitivity of SFEMG in OMG patients with simple ptosis was 91%, and the sensitivity of SFEMG in ptosis combined with diplopia was as high as 98%, with no statistically significant difference between the two. However, the sensitivity of SFEMG in OMG patients with simple diplopia was only 32%, so the analysis of the test results should be combined with the patient's clinical manifestations. A study published in 2020 showed that the ice pack test can be used as a supplementary test for SFEMG. When both the ice pack test and SFEMG are positive, the positive predictive value for OMG is as high as 95% [14].

SFEMG is not a perfect detection method. On the one hand, SFEMG abnormalities can also occur in other neuromuscular diseases, such as mitochondrial myopathy and motor neuron disease, so the analysis of the test results should be combined with the patient's clinical manifestations. On the other hand, the SFEMG examination process may be long, requiring close cooperation from the patient. Not all patients can tolerate it, and because it requires professional skills, it is not used as a routine detection method in many hospital centers, and is currently mainly used for electrophysiological research. In addition to being a useful auxiliary diagnostic tool, in most MG patients, SFEMG jitter and pulse block can also indicate the severity of the disease [15, 16]. Due to other neuromuscular diseases or technical problems, false positive results may occur [17]. However, single fiber electromyography is still the gold standard in electrophysiological tests for diagnosing MG.

8.3 Repetitive Ocular Vestibular Evoked Myogenic Potentials Is a New, Simple, Noninvasive Electrophysiological Examination

Repetitive ocular vestibular evoked myogenic potentials (RoVEMP) can detect neuromuscular transmission of extraocular muscles compared to

RNS and SFEMG [18]. The examiner places two surface electrodes on the patient's eyelids to record the myogenic activity of the inferior oblique muscle, and a ground electrode is placed on the forehead, with a frequency of 20 Hz~30 Hz. The sensitivity of the RoVEMP test for diagnosing OMG and GMG is 80% and 63%, respectively [18]. RoVEMPs can effectively distinguish MG patients from healthy controls (sensitivity 71%~89%, specificity 64%~86%) [19] and patients with other neuromuscular diseases (sensitivity 67%, specificity 82%) [18]. RoVEMP testing is fast (10~15 min), less invasive than RNS and SFEMG, and easy to operate. In patients with negative antibody detection, negative RNS results, and simple ophthalmoplegia, the RoVEMP test has significant value in the diagnosis of OMG. This noninvasive technique is a promising diagnostic tool, worthy of confirmation in further research.

8.4 Drug Therapeutic Trials

Acetylcholinesterase inhibitors (ACEIs) are the first choice of symptomatic treatment drugs for OMG. When the clinical manifestations are suspected of OMG and the antibody, electrophysiological detection, and tensilon test are all negative, the patient's myasthenia symptoms are improved after taking ACEIs, which can support the diagnosis of OMG.

8.5 Patients with Ocular Myasthenia Gravis Should Undergo Thymus Screening

The occurrence of OMG is closely related to the thymus, so all patients with OMG should undergo thymus screening to assess the thymus situation. The thymus usually degenerates before adulthood, and most MG patients may have thymus hyperplasia (up to 70%) or thymoma (10%~15%) [20]. The majority of MG patients with thymoma are AChR-Ab positive [21]. The risk of thymoma in OMG patients is 4%, and every suspected OMG patient should undergo a chest CT or MRI examination, which is very significant for deciding the next treatment plan.

8.6 New Developments in Detection Methods

MicroRNAs (miRNAs) are short endogenous noncoding RNA molecules, first discovered in the body of the nematode in 1993 [22]. Jiang et al. [23] first reported the role of MG's miRNAs. Subsequent research proposed the miRNA spectrum in serum samples or peripheral blood mononuclear cells [24]. Although the exact role of miR-30e-5p in humans needs further clarification, it is speculated that elevated levels of miR-30e-5p may reduce the expression of important proteins related to maintaining skeletal muscle homeostasis and metabolism. The sensitivity of miR-30e-5p in all OMG patients is 96%, and the sensitivity in late-onset OMG patients is 100% [24]. miR-30e-5p can serve as a potential predictive biomarker for the progression of OMG to GMG, especially for late-onset OMG patients (age ≥50 years).

References

1. Committee A Q A. American Association of Electrodiagnostic Medicine. Practice parameter for repetitive nerve stimulation and single fiber EMG evaluation of adults with suspected myasthenia gravis or Lambert-Eaton myasthenic syndrome: summary statement. Muscle Nerve. 2001;24(09):1236–8.
2. Benatar M, Kaminski H. Medical and surgical treatment for ocular myasthenia. Cochrane Database Syst Rev. 2006;12(12):CD005081.
3. Zambelis T, Kokotis P, Karandreas N. Repetitive nerve stimulation of facial and hypothenar muscles: relative sensitivity in different myasthenia gravis subgroups. Eur Neurol. 2011;65(4):203–7.
4. Howard JF. Electrodiagnosis of disorders of neuromuscular transmission. Phys Med Rehabil Clin N Am. 2013;24(1):169–92.
5. Stalberg E, Sanders D, Kouyoumdjian J. Pitfalls and errors in measuring jitter. Clin Neurophysiol. 2017;128(11):2233–41. https://doi.org/10.1016/j.clinph.2017.09.001.
6. Thornton R, Michell A. Techniques and applications of EMG: measuring motor units from structure to function. J Neurol. 2012;259(3):585–94. https://doi.org/10.1007/s00415-011-6350-0.

7. Juel V. Single fiber electromyography. Handb Clin Neurol. 2019;160:303–10. https://doi.org/10.1016/B978-0-444-64032-1.00019-9.
8. Rajasekharan C, Anishkumar V, Suresh M. Ice pack test: is it obsolete? BMJ Case Rep. 2011:bcr0420114066. https://doi.org/10.1136/bcr.04.2011.4066.
9. Vincent A, Newsom-Davis J. Acetylcholine receptor antibody as a diagnostic test for myasthenia gravis: results in 153 validated cases and 2967 diagnostic assays. Neurol Neurosurg Psychiatry. 1985;48(12):1246–52.
10. Jacobson D. Acetylcholine receptor antibodies in patients with graves' ophthalmopathy. J Neuroophthalmol. 1995;15(3):166–70.
11. Benatar M. A systematic review of diagnostic studies in myasthenia gravis. Neuromuscul Disord. 2006;16(7):459–67. https://doi.org/10.1016/j.nmd.2006.05.006.
12. Baruca M, Leonardis L, Podnar S, et al. Single fiber EMG as a prognostic tool in myasthenia gravis. Muscle Nerve. 2016;54(6):1034–40. https://doi.org/10.1002/mus.25174.
13. Giannoccaro MP, Di Stasi V, Zanesini C, et al. Sensitivity and specificity of single-fibre EMG in the diagnosis of ocular myasthenia varies accordingly to clinical presentation. J Neurol. 2020;267(3):739–45. https://doi.org/10.1007/s00415-019-09631-3.
14. Doughty CT, Guidon AC. Stronger together: diagnostic testing for ocular myasthenia gravis. Neurology. 2020; https://doi.org/10.1212/wnl.0000000000010616.
15. Konishi T, Nishitani H, Matsubara F, et al. Myasthenia gravis: relation between jitter in single-fiber EMG and antibody to acetylcholine receptor. J Neurol. 1981;31(4):386–92.
16. Sanders DB. Clinical impact of single-fiber electromyography. Muscle Nerve. 2002;11:S15–20. https://doi.org/10.1002/mus10141.
17. Okun M, Charriez C, Bhatti M, et al. Tensilon and the diagnosis of myasthenia gravis: are we using the tensilon test too much? Neurologist. 2001;7(5):295–9.
18. de Meel RHP, Keene KR, Wirth MA, et al. Repetitive ocular vestibular evoked myogenic potentials in myasthenia gravis. Neurology. 2020;94(16):e1693–701. https://doi.org/10.1212/WNL.0000000000009306.
19. Valko Y, Rosengren SM, Jung HH, et al. Ocular vestibular evoked myogenic potentials as a test for myasthenia gravis. Neurology. 2016;86(7):660–8. https://doi.org/10.1212/WNL.0000000000002383.
20. Salvi V, Gianello V, Tiberio L, et al. Cytokine targeting by miRNAs in autoimmune diseases. Front Immunol. 2019;10:15. https://doi.org/10.3389/fimmu.2019.00015.
21. Jordan B, Kellner J, Jordan K, et al. Thymic pathologies in myasthenia gravis: a preoperative assessment of CAT scan and nuclear based imaging. J Neurol. 2016;263(4):641–8. https://doi.org/10.1007/s00415-016-8023-5.
22. Lee R, Feinbaum R, Ambros V. Elegans heterochronic gene lin-4 encodes small RNAs with antisense complementarity to lin-14. Cell. 1993;75(5):843–54.
23. Jiang L, Cheng Z, Qiu S, et al. Altered let-7 expression in myasthenia gravis and let-7c mediated regulation of IL-10 by directly targeting IL-10 in Jurkat cells. Int Immunopharmacol. 2012;14(2):217–23. https://doi.org/10.1016/j.intimp.2012.07.003.
24. Sabre L, Maddison P, Wong SH, et al. miR-30e-5p as predictor of generalization in ocular myasthenia gravis. Ann Clin Transl Neurol. 2019;6(2):243–51. https://doi.org/10.1002/acn3.692.

9 Diseases Coexisting with Ocular Myasthenia Gravis

In addition to antibody detection, identifying coexisting autoimmune diseases is crucial for MG patients because they affect the progression, treatment outcomes, and mortality of the disease.

9.1 Thymoma, Optic Neuritis, Amyotrophic Lateral Sclerosis Are Highly Related to MG

Thymoma and MG are closely related, one-third of thymoma patients will develop MG. In addition, thymoma is also associated with an increased risk of certain other autoimmune diseases. The incidence of cytopenia, polymyositis, POEMS syndrome (polyneuropathy, organomegaly, endocrinopathy, monoclonal protein, and skin changes), stiff person syndrome, and autoimmune encephalitis increases in patients with thymoma, but is rare in patients with myasthenia gravis.

The incidence of neuromyelitis optica with anti-aquaporin 4 antibody (AQP4) is 40 per million [1], which has a specific connection with MG and can occur before or after the onset of MG [2].

The chance of developing amyotrophic lateral sclerosis in patients with myasthenia gravis is higher than expected in the general population. Autoimmune diseases are usually a risk factor for amyotrophic lateral sclerosis, but the correlation with myasthenia gravis is particularly strong [3, 4].

9.2 The Most Common Coexisting Disease Is Autoimmune Thyroid Disease

About 15% of MG patients will have another autoimmune disease, the most common of which is autoimmune thyroid disease, followed by systemic lupus erythematosus and rheumatoid arthritis [5]. These conditions are common in early-onset MG and MG patients with thymic hyperplasia. MG is associated with all thyroid diseases, with a greater correlation with chronic lymphocytic thyroiditis, diffuse toxic goiter, and thyrotoxicosis [6].

Graves' disease and MG may have similar pathogenesis, the Th17 cell line is involved in autoimmune thyroid disease, which may be a key factor in the occurrence of MG and Graves' disease [7]. MG patients with autoimmune thyroid disease are often associated with females, early-onset MG, and thymic hyperplasia [8]. About 10%~20% of MG patients test positive for thyroid antibodies [9]. Studies have shown that compared with other MG patients, MG patients with autoimmune thyroid disease have a milder course of disease [6, 9]. Patients with thyroid-related eye disease have hypertrophy and thickening of the extraocular muscles, causing restrictive strabismus, not paralytic strabismus. The medial rectus is the first to be affected in thyroid-related eye disease, and restrictive

Q. Zhou, J. Chen, *Ocular Myasthenia Gravis*, Experts' Perspectives on Medical Advances,
https://doi.org/10.1007/978-981-96-1245-1_9

esotropia is the most common; if exotropia occurs, coexistence with OMG should be suspected [10]. In addition to diplopia, these two diseases have very different clinical manifestations, such as thyroid-related eye disease usually has more severe symptoms when waking up in the morning, while OMG patients usually have milder symptoms when waking up in the morning [10]. The presence of comorbidities increases the difficulty of disease diagnosis, but treating thyroid disease can improve the symptoms of myasthenia gravis [11].

Due to the high prevalence of thyroid disease, it is necessary and reasonable to perform thyroid function and thyroid antibody tests on patients diagnosed with MG. Research [12] suggests the following for the evaluation of patients with ptosis and diplopia, and for MG patients with thyroid dysfunction: (1) All newly diagnosed OMG patients should be screened and treated for hyperthyroidism/hypothyroidism. (2) For any previously well-controlled myasthenia gravis patient, if the condition worsens, thyroid dysfunction should be screened. (3) In patients diagnosed with TAO, the presence of ptosis and strabismus should be evaluated for possible OMG. (4) If there are symptoms of exophthalmos, eyelid retraction, pain, or other symptoms of increased intraocular pressure, TAO should be immediately evaluated. (5) For patients with increased intraocular pressure, it is recommended to use MRI to assess whether the extraocular muscles are thickened. If thickening of the extraocular muscles is seen in the context of autoimmune disease, this will highly suggest TAO. (6) A single positive serologic, neurophysiologic test is not sufficient. Ideally, multiple testing modalities should be combined with clinical data to arrive at an accurate diagnosis. (7) Thymic hyperplasia is seen in OMG and Graves' disease, so it should not be used to distinguish between the two.

References

1. Flanagan EP, Cabre P, Weinshenker BG, et al. Epidemiology of aquaporin-4 autoimmunity and neuromyelitis optica spectrum. Ann Neurol. 2016;79(5):775–83. https://doi.org/10.1002/ana.24617.
2. Freitas E, Guimarães J. Neuromyelitis optica spectrum disorders associated with other autoimmune diseases. Rheumatol Int. 2015;35(2):243–53. https://doi.org/10.1007/s00296-014-3066-3.
3. Gotaas HT, Skeie GO, Gilhus NE. Myasthenia gravis and amyotrophic lateral sclerosis: a pathogenic overlap. Neuromusc Disord. 2016;26(6):337–41. https://doi.org/10.1016/j.nmd.2016.03.003.
4. Staff NP, Appel SH. The immune system continues to knock at the ALS door. Neuromusc Disord. 2016;26(6):335–6. https://doi.org/10.1016/j.nmd.2016.04.010.
5. Tanovska N, Novotni G, Sazdova-Burneska S, et al. Myasthenia gravis and associated diseases. Open Access Maced J Med Sci. 2018;6(3):472–8. https://doi.org/10.3889/oamjms.2018.110.
6. Lin YP, Iqbal U, Nguyen PA, et al. The concomitant association of thyroid disorders and myasthenia gravis. Transl Neurosci. 2017;8:27–30. https://doi.org/10.1515/tnsci-2017-0006.
7. Punga A, Punga T. Circulating microRNAs as potential biomarkers in myasthenia gravis patients. Ann N Y Acad Sci. 2018;1412(1):33–40. https://doi.org/10.1111/nyas.13510.
8. Kanazawa M, Shimohata T, Tanaka K, et al. Clinical features of patients with myasthenia gravis associated with autoimmune diseases. Eur J Neurol. 2007;14(12):1403–4. https://doi.org/10.1111/j.1468-1331.2007.01978.x.
9. Kubiszewska J, Szyluk B, Szczudlik P, et al. Prevalence and impact of autoimmune thyroid disease on myasthenia gravis course. Brain Behav. 2016;6(10):e00537. https://doi.org/10.1002/brb3.537.
10. Rukov JL, Wilentzik R, Jaffe I, et al. Pharmaco-miR: linking microRNAs and drug effects. Brief Bioinform. 2014;15(4):648–59. https://doi.org/10.1093/bib/bbs082.
11. Kerty E, Elsais A, Argov Z, et al. EFNS/ENS Guidelines for the treatment of ocular myasthenia. Eur J Neurol. 2014;21(5):687–93. https://doi.org/10.1111/ene.12359.
12. Claytor B, Li Y. Challenges in diagnosing coexisting ocular myasthenia gravis and thyroid eye disease. Muscle Nerve. 2020; https://doi.org/10.1002/mus.27118.

10 Differential Diagnosis of Ocular Myasthenia Gravis

10.1 Thyroid-Related Eye Disease

Thyroid-related eye disease is an autoimmune thyroid disease, characterized by self-limiting ocular muscle weakness, eyelid retraction, which can cause varying degrees of ocular muscle paralysis, and can also cause ptosis or orbicularis oculi muscle weakness, accompanied by exophthalmos or periorbital edema [1] . Orbital CT or MRI shows thickening of the extraocular muscles, hyperthyroidism or hypothyroidism, positive anti-thyroglobulin antibody, anti-thyroid peroxidase antibody, or anti-thyroid stimulating hormone receptor antibody. Thyroid eye disease and OMG can coexist.

10.2 Cranial Nerve Paralysis

Any disease that causes paralysis of cranial nerves III, IV, or VI may be confused with OMG. Intracranial mass lesions (including cavernous sinus), brainstem infarction, trauma, infection, and Miller-Fisher variant acute inflammatory demyelinating polyneuropathy can affect multiple cranial nerves, thus confusing with OMG. Cranial MRI and cerebrospinal fluid examination can help in differential diagnosis. In addition, diabetes can also cause isolated oculomotor or abducens nerve paralysis.

10.3 Other Diseases

Chronic progressive external ophthalmoplegia (CPEO) is a mitochondrial encephalomyopathy that can cause bilateral progressive non-fluctuating symmetrical ptosis and severe restriction of extraocular muscle paralysis, accompanied by proximal limb weakness. Despite severe eye muscle paralysis, diplopia usually does not exist [2] . In Kearns-Sayre syndrome (KSS), when CPEO occurs, cerebellar and/or retinal pathology related results can also be seen, combined with retinitis pigmentosa, cerebellar atrophy, and cardiac conduction block [3]. Electromyography shows myogenic damage, and a few patients may have slowed peripheral nerve conduction. Blood lactate is slightly increased; muscle biopsy and genetic testing can help confirm the diagnosis.

Oculopharyngodistal myopathy (OPDM) is an autosomal dominant inheritance with a family history; it starts in old age and manifests as progressive non-fluctuating bilateral ptosis, which may be asymmetrical. Identifying potential episodes (e.g., in old photos) can help in differential diagnosis. OPDM often finds strabismus caused by eye muscle paralysis, but no diplopia. These patients will gradually show symptoms of articulation disorders and difficulty swallowing [4]. Electromyography suggests myogenic damage. Serum creatine kinase is often normal or slightly elevated, muscle biopsy and genetic testing can help in diagnosis.

Q. Zhou, J. Chen, *Ocular Myasthenia Gravis*, Experts' Perspectives on Medical Advances,
https://doi.org/10.1007/978-981-96-1245-1_10

Myotonic dystrophy, especially type I, can cause bilateral ptosis and a certain degree of eye muscle paralysis. After scratching or tapping the muscles, there is usually a very obvious muscle stiffness, and the neck flexion and distal muscles of the lower limbs are usually weak. Other symptoms include difficulty swallowing, articulation disorders, cataracts, and arrhythmias [5].

Congenital myasthenic syndromes (CMS) are a group of rare genetic diseases caused by mutations in genes encoding NM structure and function proteins, causing NMJ transmission disorders. According to the distribution of the mutated gene-encoded protein in NMJ, CMS can be divided into presynaptic, synaptic, and postsynaptic mutations [6]. Generally, it can be distinguished by medical history and age. The clinical manifestations of CMS vary greatly and are easily misdiagnosed as antibody-negative MG, mitochondrial myopathy, etc. Symptoms such as ptosis, difficulty in opening eyes, feeding difficulties, and delayed motor development often appear at birth or in infancy. During adolescence, the eyeballs gradually become fixed, which is similar to MG in clinical and electrophysiological manifestations. The distinction mainly relies on blood stain antibody detection and whole exome sequencing. Some may appear in adulthood, similar to serum-negative MG. If the treatment is ineffective, congenital myasthenic syndrome should be considered [7].

Some congenital myopathies (such as central core disease) can manifest as prominent ophthalmoplegia and/or ptosis in adulthood. Prominent medullary symptoms are usually accompanied by external ophthalmoplegia and frequent involvement of respiratory muscles.

For patients with symptoms and signs suggestive of OMG, especially those with unclear and negative test results, it is necessary to differentiate from diseases that manifest as ptosis or external ophthalmoplegia. Careful examination of pupil function and eyelid closure is very important. If ptosis or ophthalmoplegia is accompanied by pupil involvement, oculomotor nerve palsy should be considered first rather than OMG. When eyelid closure weakness and ophthalmoplegia coexist, OMG is more often considered. Since intracranial tumors or aneurysms can produce symptoms similar to OMG by damaging the cranial nerves, cranial imaging is needed to differentiate in cases of unclear diagnosis [8]. Decompensated latent strabismus can also present similar to OMG, with patients often complaining that symptoms worsen after fatigue; however, a day-long examination fails to find fluctuating changes in eye symptoms.

References

1. Bartley GB, Gorman CA. Diagnostic criteria for Graves' ophthalmopathy. Am J Ophthalmol. 1995;119(6):792–5.
2. Richardson C, Smith T, Schaefer A, et al. Ocular motility findings in chronic progressive external ophthalmoplegia. Eye (Lond). 2005;19(3):258–63.
3. Butler IJ, Gadoth N. A review of a multisystem disorder of children and young adults. Arch Intern Med. 1976;136(11):1290–3.
4. Emery AEH. The muscular dystrophies. Lancet. 2002;359(9307):687–95.
5. Machuca-Tzili L, Brook D, Hilton-Jones D. Clinical and molecular aspects of the myotonic dystrophies: a review. Muscle Nerve. 2005;32(1):1–18.
6. Engel AG. Congenital myasthenic syndromes in 2018. Curr Neurol Neurosci Rep. 2018;18(8):1–11.
7. Garg N, Yiannikas C, Hardy TA, et al. Late presentations of congenital myasthenic syndromes: how many do we miss? Muscle Nerve. 2016;54(4):721–7.
8. Sussman J, Farrugia ME, Maddison P, et al. Myasthenia gravis: association of British neurologists' management guidelines. Pract Neurol. 2015;15(3):199–206. https://doi.org/10.1136/practneurol-2015-001126.

11 Treatment of Ocular Myasthenia Gravis

The goal of OMG treatment is to improve eye symptoms and delay or prevent the progression of OMG to GMG, reduce relapses, and minimize side effects caused by drugs.

11.1 Acetylcholinesterase Inhibitors Are the First Choice for Symptomatic Treatment of Ocular Myasthenia Gravis

Acetylcholinesterase inhibitors (ACEIs) are the first choice of symptomatic treatment drugs for OMG, used to improve myasthenic symptoms; the most commonly used is pyridostigmine which has the advantages of being safe, having a steady onset, long duration, and relatively few side effects [1], its inhibitory effect on acetylcholinesterase leads to a temporary increase in post-synaptic acetylcholine levels, but short-term side effects are common. This is caused by an increase in acetylcholine concentration at the synapses of non-neuromuscular junction toxins, resulting in side effects including gastrointestinal disorders (abdominal cramps, bloating, diarrhea, nausea), frequent urination, low blood pressure, bradycardia, sweating, salivation, tearing, increased bronchial secretions, and other symptoms of cholinergic excess. The initial dose of pyridostigmine bromide for adults starts from 30 mg, 3–4 times a day, and can gradually increase to 60–90 mg, 4–5 times a day, with the maximum dose determined by the patient's tolerance to ACEIs after medication [2]. The initial dose of pyridostigmine bromide for children is 0.5–1.0 mg/kg per day, taken 3–4 times, with a maintenance dose of 1–2 mg/kg, a maximum dose of 7 mg/kg, taken 5–6 times, often reaching peak concentration within 1–2 h [3].

ACEIs treatment helps alleviate ptosis and diplopia in most patients, but rarely completely cures [4]. Studies have found that the efficacy of ACEIs alone in treating ptosis is better than diplopia; when combined with immunosuppressants, the relief rate of diplopia is higher than using ACEIs alone [5, 6]. Previous research results suggest that ACEIs only provide symptomatic treatment and do not hinder the progression of the disease [7]. However, a study published in 2020 suggests that pyridostigmine bromide not only alleviates the symptoms of OMG, but also reduces the conversion rate of OMG to GMG [8], which may be related to the involvement of pyridostigmine bromide in immune regulation and the prevention of OMG conversion to GMG through the cholinergic anti-inflammatory pathway (CAP). Animal model results show that circulating macrophages expressing α7 nicotinic acetylcholine receptor (α7 nAChR) interact with serum acetylcholine, inhibiting the production of inflammatory cytokines including tumor necrosis factor α, high mobility group box (HMGB), and interleukin 6 (IL-6), and CAP can be terminated by red blood

Q. Zhou, J. Chen, *Ocular Myasthenia Gravis*, Experts' Perspectives on Medical Advances,
https://doi.org/10.1007/978-981-96-1245-1_11

cell-bound acetylcholinesterase [9]. Therefore, in addition to its main function, ACEIs also participate in immune regulation.

OMG is mediated by various pathogenic antibodies, and most patients require immunosuppressive therapy to achieve complete clinical remission. The most common immunosuppressants are glucocorticoids (GC), azathioprine (AZP), and mycophenolate mofetil (MMF). The 2020 version of the International Consensus Guidelines for the Management of Myasthenia Gravis [10] recommends that when anticholinesterase drugs are ineffective for ptosis or diplopia and the symptoms seriously affect the patient's quality of life, OMG patients should start hormone therapy; when hormones are ineffective, contraindicated, or intolerable, other immunosuppressants can be considered for combined use.

11.2 Corticosteroids Are the First-Line Immunotherapy for Ocular Myasthenia Gravis

Since the 1960s, GCs have remained the first-line immunotherapy drugs for OMG, regulating the production of cytokines [11], inducing T lymphocyte apoptosis [12], and inhibiting the transcription of inflammatory cytokines to reduce the production of AChR-Ab [13]. Up to 80% of OMG patients show significant improvement in symptoms after using GCs [7]. Data from a retrospective cohort study suggests that the rate of complete remission of ocular symptoms in OMG patients treated with GCs may be higher than those treated with ACEIs alone (70% vs. 21%).

The dosage of prednisone depends on the severity of ocular symptoms and the expected improvement time. For patients with mild symptoms, 10–20 mg of prednisone is taken orally daily, usually starting to improve in 2–3 weeks, significantly improving in 4–6 weeks, and showing the most noticeable improvement at 8 weeks. The dose is gradually reduced to a maintenance dose within 4–6 months, taking 0–10 mg of prednisone daily or every other day. This regimen rarely results in serious complications [14]. Medium-dose prednisone is beneficial for early relief of severe OMG symptoms, and it is recommended to use medium-dose prednisone, such as 40–60 $mg{\cdot}d^{-1}$ for 2–3 months or longer, to see significant improvement in ocular symptoms, but complete elimination of ocular symptoms may take up to a year [15]. For some OMG patients, especially those with a long duration of OMG, ocular symptoms are difficult to improve. Ozawa et al. [16] found that high-dose steroid pulse therapy has a faster onset and better therapeutic effect than oral steroids, especially for relieving diplopia symptoms. The study results show that early steroid treatment helps to reduce the conversion rate of OMG to GMG [17]. Due to the potential long-term side effects of steroid treatment, some experts suggest using steroid pulse therapy only for severe OMG patients.

The side effects of GCs include obesity, hypertension, diabetes, opportunistic infections, osteoporosis, glaucoma, cataracts, increased facial hair (in women), and gastric ulcers. These side effects usually depend on the dose and treatment duration. A low-carbohydrate, low-sodium diet can prevent or reduce weight gain; supplementing with vitamin D and bisphosphonates can help prevent osteoporosis. Even when combined with another immunosuppressant, at least one-third of patients still need long-term GC treatment to prevent disease recurrence [18, 19].

In addition to controlling symptoms, another important goal of OMG treatment is to avoid progression to GMG. Some studies have shown that early use of steroid treatment can reduce the incidence of OMG conversion to GMG [17, 20–21]. However, most conclusions are based on retrospective data and should be treated with caution. Additionally, when making treatment decisions for OMG patients, factors related to the use of GC should be considered, including antibody positivity, thymus hyperplasia, and abnormal electrophysiological tests of non-ocular muscles [22, 23, 24].

11.3 Azathioprine is the Most Commonly Used Immunosuppressant in OMG

Since the 1970s, AZP has been used as another effective immunotherapy for OMG. It is a purine analog with purine antagonist effects, interfering with DNA synthesis and hindering the proliferation of B lymphocytes and T lymphocytes. It is the most commonly used immunosuppressant in OMG [22].

Oral azathioprine is usually recommended to start at a small dose and gradually increase, with the dosage and duration determined by symptom improvement. The initial dose for children is 1–2 mg/(kg·d), and for adults it is 2–3 mg/(kg·d), taken orally 2–3 times a day; if there are no severe or intolerable adverse reactions, it can be taken long term, with a maintenance dose of 1–2 mg/(kg·d) [25]. The onset of AZP is slow, usually effective after 3–6 months of continuous use, and full effect can be reached after 1–2 years, but it has a positive effect in inhibiting disease progression [26]. AZP is usually used in conjunction with GC, significantly reducing the incidence of GMG (12%), compared to 64% in patients not treated with immunosuppressants [27], and the combined treatment effect is better than using GC alone, and can reduce the dose of GC to reduce toxic side effects [28].

Azathioprine is usually better tolerated than long-term steroid treatment [21], but careful monitoring is needed, as some side effects can be life-threatening. The main side effects include bone marrow suppression, liver damage, hair loss, flu-like symptoms, and gastrointestinal symptoms, most of which occur around 6 weeks after starting treatment. People with mutations in the thiopurine methyltransferase (TPMT) gene have a higher risk of azathioprine-induced bone marrow suppression [22]. Azathioprine increases the risk of non-melanoma skin cancer by three times [29]. Long-term use of AZA should regularly monitor the activity of TPMT to avoid potential toxicity associated with low TPMT activity, while closely monitoring blood routine and liver and kidney function. In the first month of medication, blood routine and liver and kidney function should be monitored weekly; in the first 6 months after medication, blood routine and liver and kidney function should be monitored monthly; thereafter, blood routine and liver and kidney function should be monitored every 3 months. If the white blood cell count is $<4.0 \times 10^{9}$/L, AZA should be reduced; if the white blood cell count is $<3.0 \times 10^{9}$/L or the liver function test indicator is three times the upper limit of normal, medication should be stopped immediately.

11.4 Mycophenolate Mofetil as a Second-Line Drug for the Treatment of OMG

In 2000, clinicians began using MMF in transplant patients to prevent postoperative rejection. Currently, MMF is used as a second-line drug for the treatment of OMG and can also be used in combination with steroids in the early stages. MMF is a reversible phosphatase dehydrogenase inhibitor that works by inhibiting guanosine synthesis, thereby inhibiting the replication of B lymphocytes and T lymphocytes. The starting dose of MMF is 0.5–1.0 g/d, taken orally in two doses; the maintenance dose is 1.0–1.5 g/d, and the dose should not be reduced by more than 500 mg/d per year after symptoms stabilize. Abrupt discontinuation or rapid reduction can lead to a recurrence and worsening of the disease; long-term use can enable most patients to achieve MMS or better status [30]. MMF should not be used concurrently with AZA. A prospective observational study of 31 OMG patients showed that after 4.2 years of follow-up, 87% of patients still had only ocular symptoms, suggesting that MMF plays an active role in controlling ocular symptoms and the progression of OMG to GMG [31]. MMF is safe and well tolerated in OMG patients, but a randomized controlled trial did not show any benefit of MMF in GMG [32]. Currently, there is no established recommended dose of MMF in the pediatric population [33]. MMF is teratogenic and is contraindicated in women who are planning to become pregnant or are pregnant.

The side effects of MMF are usually mild, including gastrointestinal reactions such as nausea, vomiting, diarrhea, abdominal pain, leukopenia, urinary system infections, and viral infections. Gastrointestinal discomfort is its most prominent side effect [34], and bone marrow suppression and hepatotoxicity rarely occur [22]. MMF can cause central nervous system depression, increase the risk of infection, reactivate viral infections, and increase the risk of lymphoproliferative diseases. The administration of MMF and antacids should be separated by at least 2 h, as antacids can potentially reduce the effect of MMF. Caution should be exercised when using MMF and other immunomodulators. In the first 6 months after medication, monitor blood routine and liver and kidney function every month, and thereafter every 3 months.

11.5 Cyclosporine A Is Commonly Used in Patients Who Are Poorly Responsive to or Cannot Tolerate the Side Effects of Corticosteroids and Azathioprine

Cyclosporin A (CsA) is a calcineurin phosphatase inhibitor that can block the activation of T cells and inhibit the secretion of cytokines, thereby achieving immunosuppressive effects [35]. It usually takes effect after 3–6 months of continuous use and is often used in patients who respond poorly to steroids and AZA or cannot tolerate their side effects. Early combination of CsA with steroids can significantly improve myasthenia gravis symptoms and reduce the level of AChR-Ab in the blood, but it has significant nephrotoxicity. CsA is taken orally at a dose of 2–4 mg/(kg d), and the plasma cyclosporine drug concentration should be monitored during use. The recommended blood drug concentration is 100–150 ng/mL, and the dose of cyclosporine should be adjusted based on the concentration.

Cyclosporine is contraindicated in patients with rheumatoid arthritis and psoriasis with abnormal kidney function, uncontrolled hypertension, or malignant tumors. It is a CYP3A4 inhibitor and can therefore interact with many drugs that participate in the same pathway. Patients must avoid drinking grapefruit juice as it can reduce the metabolism of cyclosporine. Statins should not be used in combination with cyclosporine as the metabolism of statins is impaired. Calcium channel blockers, carvedilol, antifungal drugs, phenytoin, phenobarbital, carbamazepine, etc. can affect the blood concentration of cyclosporine and should not be used together. When using multiple immunosuppressants, treatment should be considered. Nonsteroidal anti-inflammatory drugs should be used with caution as they can increase nephrotoxic effects; potassium-sparing diuretics should be avoided as they can enhance hyperkalemia. CsA side effects are common, including hirsutism, tremors, gum hyperplasia, and anemia, but hypertension and nephrotoxicity are the main adverse reactions limiting treatment. During medication, blood routine, liver and kidney function should be monitored at least once a month, and blood pressure should be closely monitored. CsA has been used to treat individual cases of OMG with good clinical response, but its nephrotoxicity is high and it interacts with other drugs, its side effects are significant, and it is not recommended as a first choice [36].

11.6 Tacrolimus Is the First-Choice Drug for Refractory OMG

In 2000, Japan approved tacrolimus (Tacrolimus, TAC) for the treatment of GMG that is insufficiently responsive to hormones or difficult to use due to severe side effects. In October 2009, TAC indications were extended to the treatment of OMG. TAC interferes with the signal transduction of calcineurin phosphatase, thereby inhibiting the activity of neural calcineurin phosphatase, and then inhibiting the activation of T cells and the production of various cytokines. Although TAC has a similar mechanism of action to CsA, it is better tolerated and its damage to the kidneys is less than that of CsA. It has also been proven to reduce BAFF (B-Cell Activating Factor) B cells, which are thought to play a role in pediatric OMG. Although no randomized controlled trials have been conducted, studies have shown that TAC is effective in the treatment of OMG and GMG in children. TAC is often used in MG patients who cannot tolerate the side effects of steroids and other immunosuppressants or have poor efficacy, especially in RyR-Ab positive patients. TAC takes effect quickly, generally within about 2 weeks, and the efficacy is dose-dependent. There is currently no established recommended dose of TAC in pediatric OMG patients, but one case report used 0.028 mg/kg/d as the starting dose, gradually increased after 3–4 weeks, with a target monitoring level of 5–6 ng/mL, and a maintenance dose of 0.015 mg/kg/d [37]. The maximum effect of the drug can be observed within about 1–3 months [37]. Adult TAC usage: 3.0 mg/d, taken twice on an empty stomach, or according to body weight 0.05–0.10 mg/(kg·d). It is recommended that patients screen for blood drug concentration 3–4 days after taking the drug or adjusting the dose, with an ideal drug concentration of 2–9 ng/mL [38]. In a retrospective study, TAC was used alone to treat four cases of OMG, with good clinical results [39]. A randomized, double-blind, placebo-controlled study (also including OMG patients) showed that TAC has a moderate immunosuppressive effect [40]. Yoshihiko et al. [41] showed that the combined use of TAC in the treatment of hormone-dependent OMG patients significantly improved efficacy and significantly reduced the effective dose of hormones. The most common side effects of TAC include tremors, headaches, nausea/vomiting, abdominal pain, insomnia, and tingling or swelling of the hands and feet. Tacrolimus is a CYP3A4 inhibitor, so patients should avoid grapefruit juice and any other drugs affected by this pathway. Caution should be used when other immunosuppressants are used with tacrolimus, as well as during antifungal treatment. SSRIs (except for troglitazone) can reduce the metabolism of tacrolimus and alternative treatments should be considered.

11.7 Methotrexate as a Third-Line Drug for the Treatment of OMG

Methotrexate (MTX) was produced in the 1940s. It is a folate analog that can inhibit the synthesis of purines and pyrimidines, thereby reducing T cell proliferation. MTX as a third-line drug is used for refractory or thymoma-associated MG that is ineffective with other immunosuppressants. Studies have shown that MTX has similar efficacy and tolerance to AZP and is an effective immunosuppressant [42]. Start with 10 mg of oral MTX per week, gradually increasing to 20 mg/week. If gastrointestinal adverse reactions caused by oral preparations cannot be tolerated, intramuscular injection can allow patients to tolerate higher doses [43]. It has advantages over AZP in terms of cost, weekly dosing regimen, and relatively benign side effects such as nausea and stomatitis. Elevated liver transaminases may occur, but this rarely leads to discontinuation of the drug; occasional photosensitive rash, abnormal blood count, and lung toxicity may occur. During treatment, 1 mg/d of folic acid should be added to prevent stomatitis, and close attention should be paid to side effects such as bone marrow suppression and liver damage. Methotrexate is teratogenic and is contraindicated in pregnant or planning to become pregnant women.

11.8 Rituximab May Be a Viable Option for Children with AChR-Ab Positive, Refractory Symptomatic Ocular Myasthenia Gravis

Rituximab is a monoclonal antibody against the CD20 molecule of B cells [44]. Rituximab has been used in the adult population, but there are fewer reports of its use in children with MG [45, 46]. Data shows that rituximab is effective in patients with refractory MG, such as those with persistent symptoms despite the use of multiple immunosuppressants [47]. Currently, there are no data or reports on the use of rituximab in pure OMG. However, based on published data, rituximab may be a viable option for children with AChR-Ab positive, refractory OMG. The dose of rituximab is 375 mg/m^2 as an induction dose, continued for 4 weeks. Some patients may not require a follow-up dose, but if needed, the follow-up dose is 375 mg/m^2 [34] every 4–10 months. Generally, the effect of the injection is greatest in 1 to 3 months. The most common side effects include itching, headache, dizziness, nausea/vomiting, arrhythmia, and bone marrow suppression. Rituximab may reduce the effect of live and inactivated vaccines, so it should be injected at least 2 weeks after vaccination, or 3 months after rituximab injection.

There is currently no data on the use of Eculizumab for OMG treatment. Eculizumab is a monoclonal antibody that acts as a complement inhibitor, protecting neuromuscular junctions from complement activation [48]. In 2017, the FDA approved the use of Eculizumab for the treatment of antibody-positive refractory MG [49]. In a double-blind, randomized controlled trial, AChR-Ab positive refractory GMG adult patients without thymoma showed significant improvement in myasthenia symptoms and were more able to perform daily activities after using Eculizumab [48]. Patients participating in the trial benefited after the first infusion, and the rate of MG worsening during the trial was reduced [49]. There is currently no published data on the use of Eculizumab in pediatric populations, but clinical trials are currently underway. Of all the treatments, Eculizumab is the most expensive, costing over $60,000 per month in the United States [49]. The drug is well tolerated, with the most common adverse reactions including headache, upper respiratory tract infection, nausea, and diarrhea. In one clinical trial, it was reported that patients had meningococcal sepsis. Therefore, it is recommended to vaccinate with meningococcal vaccine at least 2 weeks before infusion [48].

11.9 Intravenous Immunoglobulin and Plasma Exchange Are Short-Term Treatment Methods for Myasthenia Gravis

Intravenous immunoglobulin (IVIG) and plasmapheresis are short-term treatments and are the main means of GMG treatment. They are recommended for severe GMG patients, but not recommended for patients with pure ocular symptoms. IVIG is used for many autoimmune diseases. In MG, IVIG has been used for short-term acute treatment of myasthenic crisis, but also for monthly maintenance immunomodulatory therapy. In one study, 17 adult OMG patients used IVIG, but clinical symptoms did not significantly improve [50]. There are currently no public reports on the use of IVIG for pediatric OMG, only for pediatric GMG [51, 52]. The most common side effects of IVIG include headaches, chills, and low blood pressure, which are usually improved by reducing the infusion rate. Other side effects include renal dysfunction, aseptic meningitis, muscle spasms, allergic reactions, and thrombosis. The advantages of IVIG include rapid symptom improvement (usually within 1–2 weeks), cost-effectiveness compared to plasma exchange, and the feasibility of plasma exchange in infants and young children [34]. The initial dose or dose during myasthenic crisis can be 1 g/kg/d for two consecutive days or 0.4 g/kg/d for five consecutive days, and the maintenance dose is 0.4–2 g/kg.

There is currently no research on plasma exchange in OMG patients. It is reasonable to use intravenous immunoglobulin and plasma exchange in patients who have failed other treatments, but it must be used individually. In the case of a myasthenic crisis, plasma exchange can effectively improve muscle strength [34]. The mechanism of plasma exchange is to clear antibodies from the blood circulation, so it is an effective rapid treatment for patients who are AChR-Ab positive. The advantage of the treatment is that it usually lasts 4–10 weeks, and for those who are ineffective with other immunomodulatory treatments, it can be used as a continuous treatment [53]. Plasma exchange is usually performed five times in 8–10 days. Complications of plasma exchange include hypotension, sepsis, pneumothorax, and pulmonary embolism. The limiting factors of plasma exchange are the accessibility of treatment and the cost of services.

11.10 Thymectomy Is the Main Treatment for Thymoma OMG

Thymectomy is the main treatment for thymoma OMG. The effectiveness of thymectomy in non-thymoma OMG patients is still controversial. Two studies showed that the risk of ocular symptoms or GMG did not significantly improve after thymectomy compared to drug treatment [44, 54]. However, some researchers believe that early thymectomy can not only improve symptoms but also delay or prevent OMG from progressing to GMG [55]. A recent meta-analysis found that 50% of non-thymoma OMG patients achieved complete stable remission after thymectomy, suggesting that thymectomy is a meaningful treatment [56]. Li [57] reported that OMG patients who underwent thymectomy before progressing to GMG achieved a higher complete stable remission rate than those who underwent thymectomy after progression. In the 2020 version of the International Consensus Guidelines for the Management of Myasthenia Gravis [10], thymectomy is recommended for AChR-Ab positive OMG patients who have poor response to acetylcholinesterase inhibitors, and for OMG patients who refuse immunosuppressive treatment or have contraindications to immunosuppressive drugs. In summary, thymectomy is a method for treating thymoma and non-thymoma OMG patients, and for non-thymoma OMG patients, further multicenter randomized controlled trials are needed to determine.

11.11 Other Treatments

For patients who are difficult to treat with medication, strabismus surgery, ptosis correction surgery, occlusion therapy for amblyopia, and wearing prisms can be considered.

Studies have reported that the incidence of strabismus in children with OMG is as high as 76% [58]. All prepubescent patients with OMG will show stable ocular manifestations after the disease is fully controlled, but some patients still have residual strabismus and amblyopia [58]. Once these patients' eye positions are stable, strabismus surgery can be considered [59]. In a group of children with OMG who underwent strabismus surgery, 12 patients underwent horizontal muscle surgery combined with tendon displacement, 1 underwent vertical muscle surgery, and 5 out of 13 patients needed a second surgery [60]. This study suggests that for children with OMG whose strabismus symptoms cannot be improved by medication and whose symptoms have been stable for at least 6 months, strabismus surgery can be considered. However, this surgery carries the risk of undercorrection or overcorrection, requiring a second operation [60]. Although patients' symptoms improved after surgical intervention (9 out of 13 cases in the above study), caution should be exercised when continuing surgery, because even if the disease is stable, the degree of strabismus can continue to change [60]. The prognosis of strabismus surgery in patients with OMG is variable, and patients may need multiple surgeries, especially those who are older, have severe symptoms, and have restrictive strabismus [61]. Given the risk of postoperative recurrence and the possibility that anesthetics may exacerbate ocular symptoms, careful consideration should be given based on the actual situation.

Some patients with OMG have poor improvement in ptosis symptoms after using pyridostigmine and immunosuppressants. These patients have improved symptoms after undergoing surgery to correct ptosis, including levator muscle shortening and frontalis suspension [62, 63]. Surgical risks include exposure keratopathy, postoperative diplopia, and infection, etc. [63]. Surgical intervention to improve ptosis is more common in adult OMG, and there are no clear guidelines on when to intervene [63]. Some patients need multiple surgeries for correction. It is recommended that patients consider surgical intervention to improve ptosis only after their symptoms have been stable for at least 2 years [63].

Occlusion therapy is used to treat symptomatic diplopia and amblyopia associated with pediatric OMG. The misalignment of both eyes caused by OMG is fluctuating, which can lead to symptomatic diplopia, affecting daily work and life; monocular occlusion can solve binocular diplopia. Amblyopia is a disease of childhood, in which the connection between one or both eyes and the brain is interrupted, leading to abnormal development of vision [64]. The best time to treat amblyopia is during preschool age. If early intervention is not possible, it can lead to a worsening of amblyopia, which may require further intervention in the future, making amblyopia more difficult to treat [65].

Prisms are an effective method to improve symptoms of diplopia [60]. Prisms can correct small-angle strabismus [22, 60]. The use of prisms can be adjusted according to the changes in the disease [64].

For patients with stubborn ptosis, an eyelid brace is a cheap and noninvasive option. It is a frame glasses suitable for every patient [64]. After each frame glasses are made, it is equipped with an adjustment device according to the patient's needs to help open the eyelid. The downside is that it can easily cause dry eye syndrome and physical discomfort [64].

11.12 Treatment Progress

The treatment intervention for MG should aim to weaken the autoimmune response, enhance synaptic transmission at the neuromuscular junction, or a combination of both. A new set of treatment methods is based on the development of old, existing treatment methods. Currently, there are several main research directions in MG treatment.

11.12.1 Increase Muscle Contraction and Strengthen Neuromuscular Synaptic Transmission

EN101 is an antisense oligodeoxynucleotide that works at the mRNA level. After oral administration, the symptom improvement time is more than 24 h, which helps to increase patient compliance. Tirasemtiv is a selective activator of fast skeletal muscle troponin complex that can promote muscle contraction. Preliminary studies in MG patients have shown positive results [66], but subsequent studies have not been reported. Only a few studies have explored the possibility of strengthening neuromuscular synaptic transmission. Albuterol and ephedrine have a significant improvement effect on congenital myasthenia, and show good therapeutic effects in a small number of AChR-Ab mediated MG patients [67].

11.12.2 Regulate Autoantibody Levels

Neonatal Fc receptor (FcRn) antagonists are ideal drugs for the treatment of MG. FcRn antibodies bind to AChR-Ab and block natural lgG, causing the titer of natural IgG and AChR-Ab to drop rapidly [68]. IVIg not only inhibits pathogenic IgG, but also has multiple mechanisms of action, which may be an advantage in treating some autoimmune disease patients. Using the FcRn system to degrade specific antibodies may form an attractive research direction in the future. In fact, the principle has been proven using a novel engineered antibody-based reagent. Efgartigimod is another safe and well-tolerated FcRn antibody, which is currently undergoing phase 3 research evaluation. All patients in the Efgartigimod treatment group showed a rapid decline in total IgG and autoantibody levels, with nine patients showing rapid improvement in their condition. The correlation between the reduction in pathogenic IgG autoantibody levels and disease improvement suggests that using Efgartigimod to reduce pathogenic autoantibodies may provide an innovative treatment method [69]. Although Seldegs's research has not yet undergone clinical trials in MG patients, the ability to specifically clear antibodies against other proteins has been proven [70]. Imlifidase, based on IgG degrading enzyme, can cleave antibodies, especially IgG antibodies, and has been successfully trialed in kidney transplant patients. This drug may also be suitable for MG [71].

11.12.3 Complement Inhibitors

Complement plays a crucial role in the pathogenesis of AChR-Ab positive MG patients. Eculizumab is an inhibitor that works by inhibiting a protein, C5, that can activate complement. It has recently been approved for use in GMG, while Rituximab has been used for GMG and

OMG [72, 73]. The advantages of these drugs are that they are easily available and require small doses, but the downside is their high cost. Like IVIG and plasma exchange, it is reasonable to use these treatments in patients where other treatments have failed. Clinical trials on the therapeutic effect of another complement inhibitor, Coversini, in MG are ongoing. New complement inhibitors and FcRn blockers can be used alone or in combination to temporarily induce a rapid decrease in serum IgG in MG patients. This therapy can be used in combination with immunosuppressants to inhibit the long-term production of autoantibodies.

11.12.4 T and B Cell Therapy

The production of autoantibodies is an important cause of MG, so eliminating plasma cells that can produce autoantibodies is one effective treatment method [74]. Bortezomib is a proteasome inhibitor that can cause plasma cell apoptosis, improving the conduction speed of the postsynaptic membrane of the neuromuscular junction by inhibiting the production of AChR-Ab [75]. Studies have shown that Bortezomib can alleviate the severity of MG [76]. In addition, since helper T cells, especially Th1 and Th17, play a very important role in the pathogenesis of AChR-Ab and MuSK-Ab positive MG patients, improving the function of regulatory T cells and reducing T cell activation may become a new direction for MG treatment.

References

1. Gilhus N. Myasthenia gravis. N Engl J Med. 2016;375(26):2570–81. https://doi.org/10.1056/NEJMra1602678.
2. Fujii Y, Monden Y, Hashimoto J, et al. Acetylcholine receptor antibody-producing cells in thymus and lymph nodes in myasthenia gravis. Clin Immunol Immunopathol. 1985;34(1):141–6. https://doi.org/10.1016/0090-1229(85)90018-2.
3. Liang T, Zhi H. Progress in the treatment of childhood severe myasthenia gravis. Pediatr Pharmacy J. 2019;25(12):59–63.
4. Melzer N, Ruck T, Fuhr P, et al. Clinical features, pathogenesis, and treatment of myasthenia gravis: a supplement to the guidelines of the German Neurological Society. J Neurol. 2016;263(8):1473–94. https://doi.org/10.1007/s00415-016-8045-z.
5. Kupersmith M, Ying G. Ocular motor dysfunction and ptosis in ocular myasthenia gravis: effects of treatment. Br J Ophthalmol. 2005;89(10):1330–4. https://doi.org/10.1136/bjo.2004.063404.
6. Lee Y, Kim U. Efficacy and safety of low-to-moderate dose oral corticosteroid treatment in ocular myasthenia gravis. J Pediatr Ophthalmol Strabismus. 2018;55(5):339–42. https://doi.org/10.3928/01913913-20180620-01.
7. Evoli A, Batocchi AP, Minisci C, et al. Therapeutic options in ocular myasthenia gravis. Neuromuscul Disord. 2001;11(2):208–16.
8. Apinyawasisuk S, Chongpison Y, Thitisaksakul C, et al. Factors affecting generalization of ocular myasthenia gravis in patients with positive acetylcholine receptor antibody. Am J Ophthalmol. 2020;209:10–7. https://doi.org/10.1016/j.ajo.2019.09.019.
9. Pohanka M. Inhibitors of acetylcholinesterase and butyrylcholinesterase meet immunity. Int J Mol Sci. 2014;15(6):9809–25. https://doi.org/10.3390/ijms15069809.
10. Narayanaswami P, Sanders DB, Wolfe G, et al. International consensus guidance for management of myasthenia gravis: 2020 update. Neurology. 2020; https://doi.org/10.1212/wnl.0000000000011124.
11. Almawi W, Hess D, Rieder M. Multiplicity of glucocorticoid action in inhibiting allograft rejection. Cell Transplant. 1998;7:511–23.
12. Herold M, McPherson K, Reichardt H. Glucocorticoids in T cell apoptosis and function. Cell Mol Life Sci. 2006;63(1):60–72. https://doi.org/10.1007/s00018-005-5390-y.
13. Rogatsky I, Ivashkiv L. Glucocorticoid modulation of cytokine signaling. Tissue Antigens. 2006;68(1):1–12. https://doi.org/10.1111/j.1399-0039.2006.00599.x.
14. Kupersmith M. Does early treatment of ocular myasthenia gravis with prednisone reduce progression to generalized disease? J Neurol Sci. 2004;217(2):123–4. https://doi.org/10.1016/j.jns.2003.10.014.
15. Europa TA, Nel M, Heckmann JM. Myasthenic ophthalmoparesis: time to resolution after initiating immune therapies. Muscle Nerve. 2018;58(4):542–9. https://doi.org/10.1002/mus.26172.
16. Ozawa Y, Uzawa A, Kanai T, et al. Efficacy of high-dose intravenous methylprednisolone therapy for ocular myasthenia gravis. J Neurol Sci. 2019;402:12–5. https://doi.org/10.1016/j.jns.2019.05.003.
17. Monsul N, Patwa H, Knorr A, et al. The effect of prednisone on the progression from ocular to generalized myasthenia gravis. J Neurol Sci. 2004;217(2):131–3. https://doi.org/10.1016/j.jns.2003.08.017.
18. Benatar M, McDermott M, Sanders D, et al. Efficacy of prednisone for the treatment of ocular myasthenia (EPITOME): a randomized, controlled trial. Muscle

Nerve. 2016;53(3):363–9. https://doi.org/10.1002/mus.24769.
19. Kupersmith MJ. Ocular myasthenia gravis: treatment successes and failures in patients with long-term follow-up. J Neurol. 2009;256(8):1314–20. https://doi.org/10.1007/s00415-009-5120-8.
20. Kaminski H, Daroff R. Treatment of ocular myasthenia: steroids only when compelled. Arch Neurol. 2000;57:752–3.
21. Mee J, Paine M, Byrne E, e a. Immunotherapy of ocular myasthenia gravis reduces conversion to generalized myasthenia gravis. J Neuroophthalmol. 2003;23(4):251–5.
22. Kerty E, Elsais A, Argov Z, et al. EFNS/ENS Guidelines for the treatment of ocular myasthenia. Eur J Neurol. 2014;21(5):687–93. https://doi.org/10.1111/ene.12359.
23. Binks S, Vincent A, Palace J. Myasthenia gravis: a clinical-immunological update. J Neurol. 2016;263(4):826–34. https://doi.org/10.1007/s00415-015-7963-5.
24. Weinberg D, Rizzo J, Hayes M, et al. Ocular myasthenia gravis: predictive value of single-fiber electromyography. J Muscle nerve. 1999;22(9):1222–7.
25. Neurology Branch of Chinese Medical Association N G o C I A. China's diagnosis and treatment guidelines for myasthenia gravis 2015. In: Chinese journal of neurology; 2015. p. 934–40.
26. Lindstrom J, Seybold M, Lennon V, et al. Antibody to acetylcholine receptor in myasthenia gravis. Prevalence, clinical correlates, and diagnostic value. Neurology. 1976;26(11):1054–9.
27. Sommer N, Sigg B, Melms A, et al. Ocular myasthenia gravis: response to long-term immunosuppressive treatment. J Neurol Neurosurg Psychiatry. 1997;62(2):156–62.
28. Palace J, Newsom-Davis J, Lecky B. A randomized double-blind trial of prednisolone alone or with azathioprine in myasthenia gravis. Myasthenia gravis study group. J Neurol. 1998;50(6):1778–83.
29. Pedersen EG, Pottegard A, Hallas J, et al. Risk of non-melanoma skin cancer in myasthenia patients treated with azathioprine. Eur J Neurol. 2014;21(3):454–8. https://doi.org/10.1111/ene.12329.
30. Chan J. Mycophenolate mofetil for ocular myasthenia. J Neurol. 2008;255(4):510–3. https://doi.org/10.1007/s00415-008-0718-9.
31. Sanders D, Wolfe G, Narayanaswami P. Developing treatment guidelines for myasthenia gravis. Ann N Y Acad Sci. 2018;1412(1):95–101. https://doi.org/10.1111/nyas.13537.
32. Sanders DB, Hart IK, Mantegazza R, et al. An international, phase III, randomized trial of mycophenolate mofetil in myasthenia gravis. Neurology. 2008;71(6):400–6. https://doi.org/10.1212/01.wnl.0000312374.95186.cc.
33. Aricha R, Mizrachi K, Fuchs S, et al. Blocking of IL-6 suppresses experimental autoimmune myasthenia gravis. J Autoimmun. 2011;36(2):135–41. https://doi.org/10.1016/j.jaut.2010.12.001.
34. O'Connell K, Ramdas S, Palace J. Management of juvenile myasthenia gravis. Front Neurol. 2020;11:743. https://doi.org/10.3389/fneur.2020.00743.
35. Halloran P, Kung L, Noujaim J. Calcineurin and the biological effect of cyclosporine and tacrolimus. Transplant Proc. 1998;30(5):2167–70.
36. Ciafaloni E, Nikhar N, Massey J, et al. Retrospective analysis of the use of cyclosporine in myasthenia gravis. Neurology. 2000;55(3):448–50. https://doi.org/10.1212/wnl.55.3.448.
37. Ishigaki K, Shishikura K, Murakami T, et al. Benefits of FK 506 for refractory eye symptoms in a young child with ocular myasthenia gravis. Brain Dev. 2009;31(8):634–7. https://doi.org/10.1016/j.braindev.2008.08.016.
38. Chang T. Chinese guidelines for diagnosis and treatment of myasthenia gravis (2020 edition). Chinese J Neuroimmunol Neurol. 2021;28(01):1–12.
39. Yagi Y, Sanjo N, Yokota T, et al. Tacrolimus monotherapy: a promising option for ocular myasthenia gravis. Eur Neurol. 2013;69(6):344–5. https://doi.org/10.1159/000347068.
40. Yoshikawa H, Kiuchi T, Saida T, et al. Randomised, double-blind, placebo-controlled study of tacrolimus in myasthenia gravis. J Neurol Neurosurg Psychiatry. 2011;82(9):970–7. https://doi.org/10.1136/jnnp-2011-300148.
41. Isshiki Y, Mimura O, Gomi F. Clinical features and treatment status of antiacetylcholine receptor antibody-positive ocular myasthenia gravis. Jpn J Ophthalmol. 2020; https://doi.org/10.1007/s10384-020-00770-z.
42. Heckmann J, Rawoot A, Bateman K, et al. A single-blinded trial of methotrexate versus azathioprine as steroid-sparing agents in generalized myasthenia gravis. BMC Neurol. 2011;11:97.
43. Pasnoor M, He J, Herbelin L, et al. A randomized controlled trial of methotrexate for patients with generalized myasthenia gravis. Neurology. 2016;87(1):57–64. https://doi.org/10.1212/wnl.0000000000002795.
44. Sanders DB, Evoli A. Immunosuppressive therapies in myasthenia gravis. Autoimmunity. 2010;43(5-6):428–35. https://doi.org/10.3109/08916930903518107.
45. Wylam ME, Anderson PM, Kuntz NL, et al. Successful treatment of refractory myasthenia gravis using rituximab: a pediatric case report. J Pediatr. 2003;143(5):674–7.
46. Tzaribachev N, Koetter I, Kuemmerle-Deschner JB, et al. Rituximab for the treatment of refractory pediatric autoimmune diseases: a case series. Cases J. 2009;2:6609. https://doi.org/10.1186/1757-1626-0002-0000006609.
47. Zebardast N, Patwa HS, Novella SP, et al. Rituximab in the management of refractory myasthenia gra-

vis. Muscle Nerve. 2010;41(3):375–8. https://doi.org/10.1002/mus.21521.
48. Dhillon S. Eculizumab: a review in generalized myasthenia gravis. Drugs. 2018;78(3):367–76. https://doi.org/10.1007/s40265-018-0875-9.
49. Edmundson C, Guidon AC. Eculizumab: a Complementary addition to existing long-term therapies for myasthenia gravis. Muscle Nerve. 2019;60(1):7–9. https://doi.org/10.1002/mus.26512.
50. Zinman L, Ng E, Bril V. IV immunoglobulin in patients with myasthenia gravis: a randomized controlled trial. Neurology. 2007;68(11):837–41.
51. VanderPluym J, Vajsar J, Jacob FD, et al. Clinical characteristics of pediatric myasthenia: a surveillance study. Pediatrics. 2013;132(4):e939–44. https://doi.org/10.1542/peds.2013-0814.
52. Selcen D, Dabrowski ER, Michon AM, et al. High-dose intravenous immunoglobulin therapy in juvenile myasthenia gravis. Pediatr Neurol. 2000;22(1):40–3.
53. Andrews PI. Autoimmune myasthenia gravis in childhood. Semin Neurol. 2004;24(1):101–10.
54. Al-Haidar M, Benatar M, Kaminski H. Ocular myasthenia. Neurol Clin. 2018;36(2):241–51. https://doi.org/10.1016/j.ncl.2018.01.003.
55. Mineo TC, Ambrogi V. Outcomes after thymectomy in class I myasthenia gravis. J Thorac Cardiovasc Surg. 2013;145(5):1319–24. https://doi.org/10.1016/j.jtcvs.2012.12.053.
56. Yang HW, Wang YX, Bao J, et al. Correlation of HLA-DQ and TNF-α gene polymorphisms with ocular myasthenia gravis combined with thyroid-associated ophthalmopathy. Biosci Rep. 2017;37(2) https://doi.org/10.1042/bsr20160440.
57. Li F, Li Z, Chen Y, et al. Thymectomy in ocular myasthenia gravis before generalization results in a higher remission rate. Eur J Cardiothorac Surg. 2020;57(3):478–87. https://doi.org/10.1093/ejcts/ezz275.
58. Ortiz S, Borchert M. Long-term outcomes of pediatric ocular myasthenia gravis. Ophthalmology. 2008;115(7)
59. Peragallo JH, Velez FG, Demer JL, et al. Long-term follow-up of strabismus surgery for patients with ocular myasthenia gravis. J Neuro-ophthalmol. 2013;33(1):40–4. https://doi.org/10.1097/WNO.0b013e318280d630.
60. Park K-A, Oh SY. Treatment for diplopia in patients with myasthenia gravis. Graefe's Arch Clin Exp Ophthalmol. 2013;251(3):895–901. https://doi.org/10.1007/s00417-012-2227-x.
61. Wong SH, Petrie A, Plant GT. Ocular myasthenia gravis: toward a risk of generalization score and sample size calculation for a randomized controlled trial of disease modification. J Neuroophthalmol. 2016;36(3):252–8.
62. Bradley EA, Bartley GB, Chapman KL, et al. Surgical correction of blepharoptosis in patients with myasthenia gravis. Ophthalmic Plast Reconstr Surg. 2001;17(2):103–10.
63. Brogan K, Farrugia ME, Crofts K. Ptosis surgery in patients with myasthenia gravis: a useful adjunct to medical therapy. Semin Ophthalmol. 2018;33(3):429–34. https://doi.org/10.1080/08820538.2017.1284871.
64. Belliveau MJ, Oestreicher JH. Ptosis repair in ocular myasthenia gravis. Semin Ophthalmol. 2017;32(5):564–8. https://doi.org/10.3109/08820538.2015.1131835.
65. Han J, Han SY, Han S-H, et al. Strabismus surgery and long-term visual outcomes in patients with pre-adolescent onset ocular myasthenia gravis. Graefe's Arch Clin Exp Ophthalmol. 2015;253(1):157–63. https://doi.org/10.1007/s00417-014-2847-4.
66. Sanders D, Rosenfeld J, Dimachkie M, et al. A double-blinded, randomized, placebo-controlled trial to evaluate efficacy, safety, and tolerability of single doses of tirasemtiv in patients with acetylcholine receptor-binding antibody-positive myasthenia gravis. Neurotherapeutics. 2015;12(2):455–60. https://doi.org/10.1007/s13311-015-0345-y.
67. Lee M, Beeson D, Palace J. Therapeutic strategies for congenital myasthenic syndromes. Ann N Y Acad Sci. 2018;1412(1):129–36. https://doi.org/10.1111/nyas.13538.
68. Ulrichts P, Guglietta A, Dreier T, et al. Neonatal Fc receptor antagonist efgartigimod safely and sustainably reduces IgGs in humans. J Clin Invest. 2018;128(10):4372–86.
69. JF H Jr, Bril V, Burns TM, et al. Randomized phase 2 study of FcRn antagonist efgartigimod in generalized myasthenia gravis. Neurology. 2019;92(23):e2661–73. https://doi.org/10.1212/WNL.0000000000007600.
70. Devanaboyina S, Khare P, Challa D, et al. Engineered clearing agents for the selective depletion of antigen-specific antibodies. Nat Commun. 2017;8:15314. https://doi.org/10.1038/ncomms15314.
71. Lonze BE, Tatapudi VS, Weldon EP, et al. IdeS (Imlifidase): a novel agent that cleaves human IgG and permits successful kidney transplantation across high-strength donor-specific antibody. Ann Surg. 2018;268(3):488–96. https://doi.org/10.1097/SLA.0000000000002924.
72. Howard JF, Utsugisawa K, Benatar M, et al. Safety and efficacy of eculizumab in anti-acetylcholine receptor antibody-positive refractory generalised myasthenia gravis (REGAIN): a phase 3, randomised, double-blind, placebo-controlled, multicentre study. Lancet Neurol. 2017;16(12):976–86. https://doi.org/10.1016/s1474-4422(17)30369-1.
73. Iorio R, Damato V, Alboini PE, et al. Efficacy and safety of rituximab for myasthenia gravis: a systematic review and meta-analysis. J Neurol. 2015;262(5):1115–9. https://doi.org/10.1007/s00415-014-7532-3.
74. Hiepe F, Radbruch A. Plasma cells as an innovative target in autoimmune disease with renal manifestations. Nat Rev Nephrol. 2016;12(4):232–40. https://doi.org/10.1038/nrneph.2016.20.

75. Gomez A, Vrolix K, Martinez-Martinez P, et al. Proteasome inhibition with bortezomib depletes plasma cells and autoantibodies in experimental autoimmune myasthenia gravis. J Immunol. 2011;186(4):2503–13. https://doi.org/10.4049/jimmunol.1002539.

76. Gomez A, Willcox N, Vrolix K, et al. Proteasome inhibition with bortezomib depletes plasma cells and specific autoantibody production in primary thymic cell cultures from early-onset myasthenia gravis patients. J Immunol. 2014;193(3):1055–63. https://doi.org/10.4049/jimmunol.1301555.

12 International Consensus Guidelines for Myasthenia Gravis Management: 2020 Update

12.1 Theme of Ocular Myasthenia Gravis Treatment

In November 2020, the Myasthenia Gravis Foundation of America (MGFA), the MGFA has released the "International Consensus Guidelines for the Management of Myasthenia Gravis: 2020 Update" [1] , which updates some treatment content, including the treatment theme of OMG. This book provides an overview of the newly added treatment theme of OMG in the 2020 update for clinical doctors to refer to.

The 2016 version did not distinguish between OMG and GMG when discussing the symptoms of myasthenia gravis and immunosuppressive treatment. The 2020 update treats OMG as an independent chapter and proposes the concept of early treatment, which is based on the results of a series of clinical studies of OMG or including OMG subgroup analysis.

Recommendation 1: Cholinesterase inhibitors are the first choice for symptomatic treatment of OMG. If symptomatic treatment is ineffective and extraocular muscle paralysis leads to functional limitations or symptoms trouble the patient, immunosuppressive treatment should be initiated.

Recommendation 2: The initial immunosuppressive treatment for OMG should use corticosteroid. If single treatment is ineffective or there are contraindications or intolerance to hormones, other non-hormonal immunosuppressive drugs can be added.

Recommendation 3: Evidence from a small-scale randomized controlled trial published in 2016 suggests that low-dose hormone treatment is effective for OMG, and it is recommended to initially use low-dose hormones to avoid the side effects of high-dose hormones [2] . This single-center small-scale randomized controlled study included 11 OMG patients who did not achieve the minimum therapeutic effect after 4–6 weeks of bromopride treatment. They were divided into six cases in the prednisone group and five cases in the placebo group. The results showed that five cases (83%) in the prednisone group achieved therapeutic effects after 14 weeks of prednisone treatment (median dose of 15 mg/d), and none in the placebo group achieved the minimum therapeutic effect. Subsequently, three cases in the placebo group received prednisone treatment (60 mg/d, rapid reduction), of which two cases achieved therapeutic effects.

Recommendation 4: It is recommended that for OMG, especially AChR-Ab positive OMG patients, if symptomatic treatment is ineffective and refusal to use immunosuppressants or there are contraindications to immunosuppressive treatment, or if immunosuppressive treatment is ineffective, thymectomy can be considered.

Q. Zhou, J. Chen, *Ocular Myasthenia Gravis*, Experts' Perspectives on Medical Advances,
https://doi.org/10.1007/978-981-96-1245-1_12

References

1. Narayanaswami P, Sanders DB, Wolfe G, et al. International consensus guidance for management of myasthenia gravis: 2020 update. Neurology. 2020; https://doi.org/10.1212/wnl.0000000000011124.
2. Halloran P, Kung L, Noujaim J. Calcineurin and the biological effect of cyclosporine and tacrolimus. Transplant Proc. 1998;30(5):2167–70.

13 Risk of Ocular Myasthenia Gravis Transitioning to Generalized Myasthenia Gravis

13.1 The Clinical Course and Risk Factors in the First Three Years Are Crucial for Prognosis

In recent years, a series of studies have shown that the proportion of OMG patients transitioning to GMG is relatively low, about 18–20% [1, 2], which may be related to the early diagnosis and treatment of patients with mild symptoms. About 10–14% of OMG patients recover without treatment [3, 4]. The clinical course of the first three years is crucial in determining the prognosis of the disease [4].

Giuliana [5] and others conducted a cohort study on 175 patients with OMG, and found that during the observation period (median 83 months, range 24–158 months), 37 patients (21.1%) progressed to GMG, of which 23 were women (62%). The probabilities of OMG patients with positive MuSK-Ab, positive AChR-Ab, and seronegative converting to GMG were 75%, 26.2%, and 13.7%, respectively, indicating that gender, positive AChR-Ab, and positive MuSK-Ab are independent risk factors for conversion to GMG. MG patients with positive MuSK-Ab have a much higher risk of systemic symptoms than those with positive AChR-Ab; seronegative OMG patients have a lower risk of converting to GMG [5, 6]. A retrospective cohort study of 101 OMG patients (who did not receive any form of immunosuppressive treatment) identified significant predictive factors including serological positivity, thymic hyperplasia, and comorbidities including other autoimmune diseases [7]. A retrospective analysis of 223 OMG patients who received immunosuppressive treatment found that age of onset, disease course, and facial nerve RNS test can predict the conversion of OMG to GMG under immunosuppressive treatment [8].

Electrophysiological evidence of subclinical GMG has been considered a risk factor for the progression of OMG to GMG. A prospective study of 39 OMG patients within 4 months of onset showed that abnormalities in the extensor digitorum SFEMG are common, occurring in 70% of patients. The proportion of OMG patients with abnormal SFEMG converting to GMG is higher than those with normal SFEMG (57% vs. 18%) [9]. A subsequent large-scale retrospective study confirmed the high incidence of SFEMG abnormalities in OMG patients (68–82%), indicating that SFEMG has no predictive value for the risk of conversion to GMG [10, 11].

If OMG patients do not convert to GMG, their clinical course is often benign, and ocular symptoms usually peak in severity within 1–3 years [12]. In a retrospective analysis of 78 cases of OMG, 54 remained with only ocular symptoms during the follow-up period (average time 8.3 years); among these patients, 54% achieved complete clinical remission, [13]. However, the quality of life of patients who did not reach the mildest symptoms declined, and more severe ocular symptoms at onset suggest the possibility of adverse reactions to treatment may increase [14].

Q. Zhou, J. Chen, *Ocular Myasthenia Gravis*, Experts' Perspectives on Medical Advances,
https://doi.org/10.1007/978-981-96-1245-1_13

References

1. Peeler CE, De Lott LB, Nagia L, et al. Clinical utility of acetylcholine receptor antibody testing in ocular myasthenia gravis. JAMA Neurol. 2015;72(10):1170–4. https://doi.org/10.1001/jamaneurol.2015.1444.
2. Mazzoli M, Ariatti A, Valzania F, et al. Factors affecting outcome in ocular myasthenia gravis. Int J Neurosci. 2018;128(1):15–24. https://doi.org/10.1080/00207454.2017.1344237.
3. Ishigaki K, Shishikura K, Murakami T, et al. Benefits of FK 506 for refractory eye symptoms in a young child with ocular myasthenia gravis. Brain Dev. 2009;31(8):634–7. https://doi.org/10.1016/j.braindev.2008.08.016.
4. Grob D, Arsura E, Brunner N, et al. The course of myasthenia gravis and therapies affecting outcome. Ann N Y Acad Sci. 1987;505:472–99.
5. Galassi G, Mazzoli M, Ariatti A, et al. Antibody profile may predict outcome in ocular myasthenia gravis. Acta Neurol Belg. 2018;118(3):435–43. https://doi.org/10.1007/s13760-018-0943-7.
6. Gilhus N. Myasthenia gravis. N Engl J Med. 2016;375(26):2570–81. https://doi.org/10.1056/NEJMra1602678.
7. Wong SH, Petrie A, Plant GT. Ocular myasthenia gravis: toward a risk of generalization score and sample size calculation for a randomized controlled trial of disease modification. J Neuroophthalmol. 2016;36(3):252–8.
8. Ding JQ, Zhao SJ, Ren KX, et al. Prediction of generalization of ocular myasthenia gravis under immunosuppressive therapy in Northwest China. BMC Neurol. 2020;20(1) https://doi.org/10.1186/s12883-020-01805-1.
9. Weinberg D, Rizzo J, Hayes M, et al. Ocular myasthenia gravis: predictive value of single-fiber electromyography. J Muscle nerve. 1999;22(9):1222–7.
10. Rostedt A, Saders LL, Edards LJ, et al. Predictive value of single-fiber electromyography in the extensor digitorum communis muscle of patients with ocular myasthenia gravis: a retrospective study. J Clin Neuromuscul Dis. 2000;2(1):6–9. https://doi.org/10.1097/00131402-200009000-00003.
11. Guan YZ, Cui LY, Liu MS, et al. Single-fiber electromyography in the extensor digitorum communis for the predictive prognosis of ocular myasthenia gravis: a retrospective study of 102 cases. Chin Med J. 2015;128(20):2783–6. https://doi.org/10.4103/0366-6999.167354.
12. Grob D, Brunner N, Namba T, et al. Lifetime course of myasthenia gravis. Muscle Nerve. 2008;37(2):141–9. https://doi.org/10.1002/mus.20950.
13. Sanders DB, Evoli A. Immunosuppressive therapies in myasthenia gravis. Autoimmunity. 2010;43(5-6):428–35. https://doi.org/10.3109/08916930903518107.
14. Suzuki S, Murai H, Imai T, et al. Quality of life in purely ocular myasthenia in Japan. BMC Neurol. 2014;14(01):142.

14 Difficult Case Analysis

14.1 A Case of Ocular Myasthenia Gravis Misdiagnosed as Right Eye Double Superior Rectus Palsy

The patient is a 17-year-old male who sought surgical improvement for his drooping right upper eyelid at the First Affiliated Hospital of Jinan University's Ophthalmology Department on August 17, 2020. The patient's family reported that the right eye ptosis appeared shortly after birth and was not treated. The drooping right upper eyelid is now affecting his vision and appearance, so he came to our hospital's ophthalmology outpatient clinic for further diagnosis and treatment. He denies any birth trauma, eye trauma, surgical history, or similar eye diseases in the family. Ophthalmic examination: Right eye uncorrected visual acuity: +1.7 logMAR, corrected visual acuity: +5.50 DS/−0.75 DC*130°→ +0.5 logMAR, left eye uncorrected visual acuity: +0.2 logMAR, corrected visual acuity: +1.25DS/−0.50DC*160°→ 0 logMAR. The right upper eyelid droops, covering half of the pupil (Fig. 14.1a). The right palpebral fissure height is 3 mm, and when the left eye is covered, the right palpebral fissure height increases to 7 mm (Fig. 14.1b); the levator muscle strength is 5 mm, and the frontalis muscle strength is 8 mm; the left palpebral fissure height is 9 mm, the levator muscle strength is 10 mm, and the frontalis muscle strength is 10 mm. Hirschberg test: when looking straight ahead, the right eye is tilted downward by 15°. Eye movement examination: the right eye's upward movement is completely restricted in the nasal and temporal directions (Fig. 14.2), the left eye's eye movement is normal, and there is no compensatory head position. Prism examination: When the left eye is looking horizontally at a 33 cm target, the right eye is down by 35PD. The MRI results of the orbit and optic nerve show no obviousnn abnormalities. The outpatient clinic diagnosed "right eye double elevator palsy" and admitted him to the hospital. After admission, it was found that the patient's right eye ptosis exhibited a pattern of being milder in the morning and worsening in the evening. Considering the past medical history and the fluctuating clinical manifestations of the right eye ptosis, it is considered to be ocular myasthenia gravis in children, so relevant examinations for ocular myasthenia gravis were carried out. Examination results: Neostigmine test (+) (Fig. 14.3), fatigue test (+) (Fig. 14.4), acetylcholine receptor antibody (+), repetitive nerve stimulation (−). Thyroid ultrasound: The size of the bilateral thyroid is normal, and the changes in the echo and blood flow inside it suggest a high possibility of a colloid cyst; no obvious abnormalities were found in the orbital MRI and chest CT. Combined with the medical history, clinical manifestations, and laboratory examinations, it was diagnosed as ocular myasthenia gravis in children. He was discharged with

Q. Zhou, J. Chen, *Ocular Myasthenia Gravis*, Experts' Perspectives on Medical Advances,
https://doi.org/10.1007/978-981-96-1245-1_14

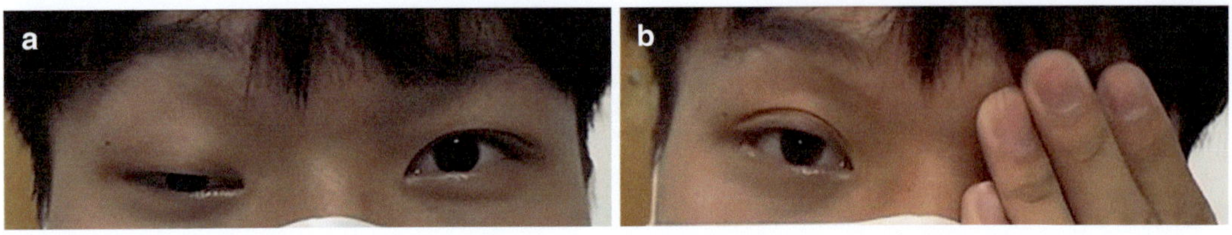

Fig. 14.1 Binocular eye position and monocular eye position of right eye. (**a**) The patient has right eyelid ptosis covering half of the pupil along with 15° of downward deviation, and no obvious upper eyelid drooping in the left eye. (**b**) The patient's right upper eyelid drooping is lessening when the left eye is covered

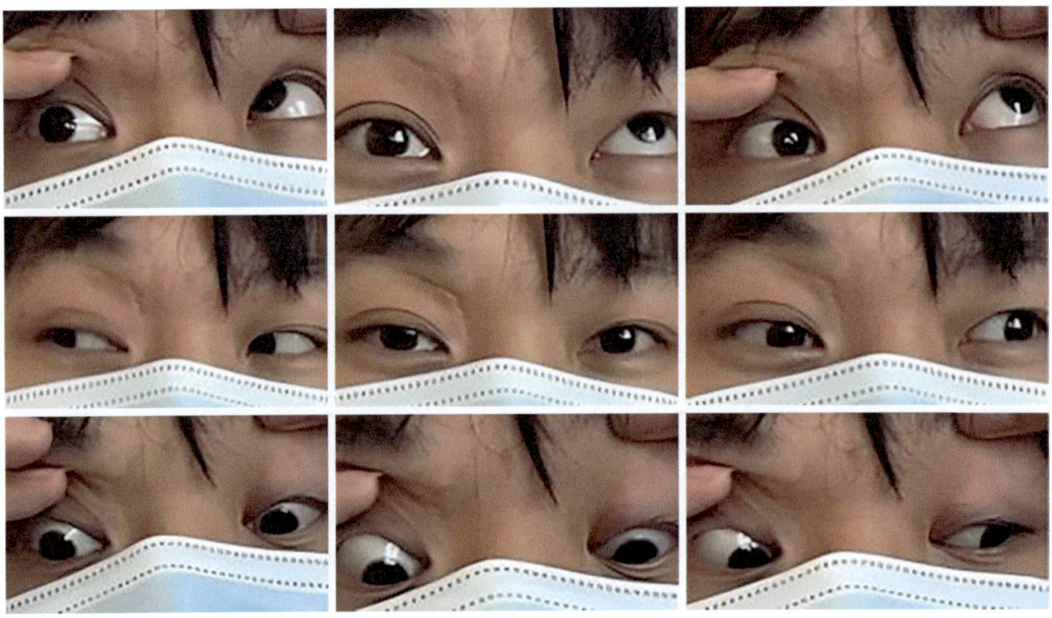

Fig. 14.2 Nine positions diagram of both eyes
When looking up, the right eye's upward movement in the nasal and temporal directions is restricted completely, and the left eye's upward movement is in place

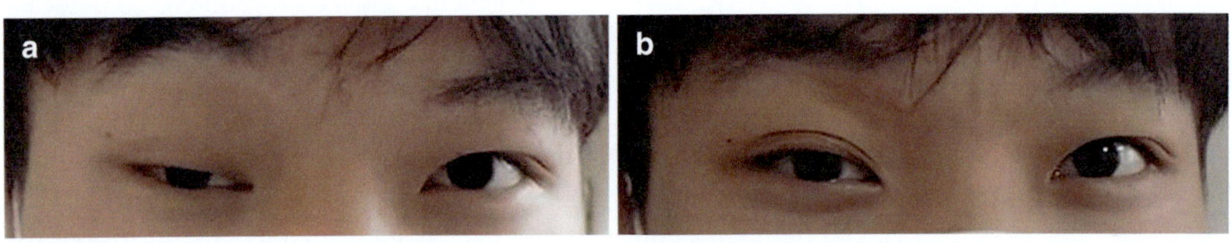

Fig. 14.3 Comparison of the patient'' right ptosis with downward deviation before and after the Neostigmine test. (**a**) Shows the obvious right eye downward deviation accompanied by upper eyelid drooping before the Neostigmine test. (**b**) Shows the obvious improvement of the right eye downward deviation and upper eyelid drooping after the Neostigmine test

pyridostigmine bromide combined with a small dose of prednisone acetate for treatment. One week later, the right palpebral fissure increased to 9 mm (Fig. 14.5).

[Case Analysis]

This is a case of a patient who was misdiagnosed with double elevator palsy instead of ocular myasthenia gravis in children.

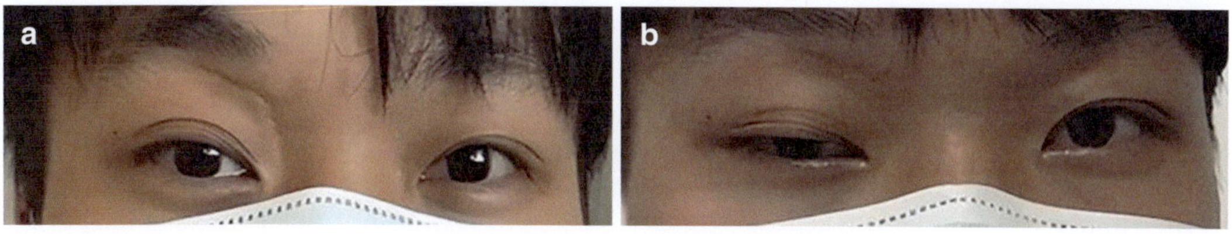

Fig. 14.4 Comparison of ptosis of right eye in the morning and in the afternoon. (**a**) Before fatigue (morning), the right eyelid ptosis is not obvious. (**b**) After fatigue (afternoon), the right eyelid ptosis is more obvious than in the morning

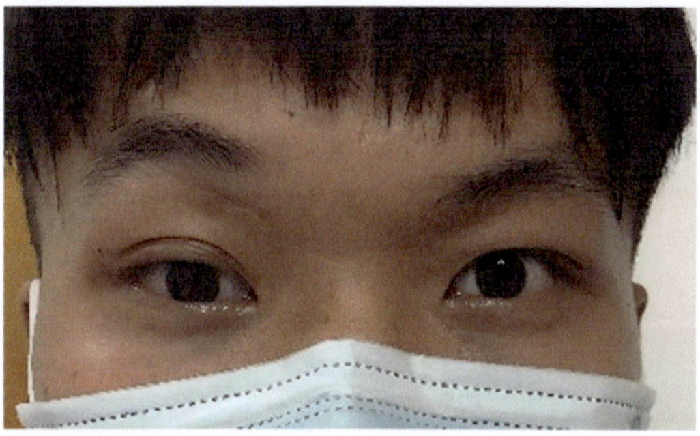

Fig. 14.5 The appearance of both eyes after 1 week of treatment
One week after treatment, the right eyelid ptosis and hypotropia have significantly improved

Double elevator palsy (DEP) is a relatively rare ocular motor disorder with an unclear etiology, characterized by simultaneous paralysis of the superior rectus and inferior oblique muscles of one eye [1]. Clinically, it presents as hypotropia and pseudoptosis of the affected eye when the non-paralyzed eye is fixating. Pseudoptosis may mask the true vertical strabismus, leading clinicians to misdiagnose it as congenital ptosis and then perform ptosis correction surgery [1]. In this case, when the patient's left eye was fixating, the right eye showed hypotropia with ptosis; when the left eye was covered, the ptosis of the right eye improved; this suggested pseudoptosis, thus ruling out the diagnosis of congenital ptosis. The patient's initial examination was consistent with DEP, and surgery is the only treatment for DEP, so the outpatient clinic planned to admit the patient for strabismus correction surgery for "right eye double elevator palsy." After admission, it was found that the right eyelid ptosis showed a characteristic of being lighter in the morning and heavier in the evening, highly suggestive of ocular myasthenia gravis in children. A series of tests related to ocular myasthenia gravis were performed. The diagnosis of OMG was confirmed based on the characteristic of the right eyelid ptosis being lighter in the morning and heavier in the evening, positive neostigmine test, and positive acetylcholine receptor antibody.

The forms of extraocular muscle paralysis in MG are diverse and can involve both elevators (superior rectus and inferior oblique) [2]. Ptosis can occur unilaterally or bilaterally, and sometimes alternates between the left and right. A recent study found that 59% of patients presented with bilateral asymmetric ptosis, 27% of patients presented with unilateral ptosis, and only 4% of patients presented with bilateral symmetric ptosis [3]. The early symptoms of OMG are similar to other diseases and are often misdiagnosed as cranial nerve palsy, eyelid spasm, motor neuron disease, etc. [4].

Ocular myasthenia gravis in children is OMG that begins in childhood. Foreign studies show that 10–15% of MG patients each year are children, and OMG accounts for about 27–93% of pediatric MG [5]. In China, the incidence of juvenile myasthenia gravis (JMG) is as high as 50%; it is mainly OMG [6]. This indicates that there is a significant racial difference in juvenile OMG. Most OMG children present with ptosis and/or strabismus, with exotropia being the most common [7]. Unlike adult OMG, juvenile OMG rarely transforms into generalized MG, and the complete remission rate is high. Even if the symptoms are not completely relieved, the ocular symptoms are stable [7]. The patient in this case had been ill since childhood and was still diagnosed with ocular myasthenia gravis, and had not yet transformed into GMG, which further demonstrated the above view that juvenile OMG rarely transforms into generalized MG.

There is a great risk of misdiagnosing OMG as bilateral superior rectus palsy. On the one hand, the primary disease is not treated in time, which will accelerate the patient's progression to generalized myasthenia gravis, seriously endangering the quality of life and even the life of the patient; on the other hand, due to the fluctuating ocular symptoms of OMG patients, even if the condition is stable, the degree of strabismus can continue to change after surgery, greatly increasing the risk of doctor-patient conflict. Considering the risk of postoperative recurrence and the possibility of anesthesia drugs aggravating ocular symptoms, it should be carefully considered according to the actual situation.

For any form of unilateral or bilateral ptosis, diplopia, or ocular muscle paralysis, OMG should be considered for evaluation [8]. This case reminds the majority of clinical ophthalmologists that when patients present with ptosis and ocular muscle involvement, OMG must be ruled out. At the initial diagnosis, the focus should be on observing and asking whether the patient's ocular manifestations have the characteristics of fluctuation, lighter in the morning and heavier in the evening, worsening after activity, and alleviating during rest, so as not to miss or misdiagnose and cause serious harm to the patient's quality of life or even life.

14.2 A Case of Misdiagnosis of Thyroid-Related Eye Disease Combined with Ocular Myasthenia Gravis

The patient is a 47-year-old male who visited the Ophthalmology Outpatient Clinic of the First Affiliated Hospital of Jinan University on 2020-05-29 due to "double vision and left eye hypertropia for 2 months." The patient has had Graves' disease for half a year and is currently undergoing drug treatment. Eye examination: naked eye vision right eye +0.3 logMAR, left eye +0.2 logMAR. Both eyes have ptosis, with the upper eyelid margin covering one-third of the corneal margin. Both eyeballs are slightly protruding, with the right eye protruding 18 mm and the left eye 17 mm. Left eye hypertropia about 35° (Fig. 14.6A1), left eye downward movement limited -4 (Fig. 14.6A2). Imaging examination for diplopia: vertical diplopia, the largest diplopia distance is to the lower left, and the peripheral image is the left eye. Orbital MRI showed (Fig. 14.7): thickening of the left eye's medial rectus, lateral rectus, and inferior rectus, and the right eye's lateral rectus. Denies history of diabetes, coronary heart disease, etc. denies history of head and eye trauma, denies other surgical history, denies family history of genetic diseases. After admission, it was found that the double vision and left eye hypertropia showed the characteristics of being lighter in the morning and heavier in the evening. Combined with the orbital MRI examination suggesting that the left eye's inferior rectus muscle belly was thickened, which was inconsistent with the manifestation of the affected eye's downward movement limitation, it was considered to be thyroid-related eye disease combined with ocular myasthenia gravis, so the relevant examination of ocular myasthenia gravis was performed. The neostigmine test was positive (Fig. 14.6B1/B2), and the ELISA method detected that the concentration of acetylcholine receptor antibodies was 17.94 nmol/L↑ (normal value <0.45 nmol/L). Thyroid examination: thyrotropin receptor antibody: >998.00 IU/L (normal value 0–9 IU/L); Free triiodothyronine is 15.67 pmol/L↑ (normal value 3.09–7.42 pmol/L), serum total triiodothyronine is 4.82 pmol/L↑ (normal value 1.01–2.48 pmol/L), free thyroxine is 44.38 pmol/L↑ (normal value 7.64–16.03 pmol/L), serum total thyroxine is 19.15 nmol/L↑ (normal value 69.97–152.52 nmol/L), thyroid-stimulating hormone is 0.001 mIU/L↓ (normal value 0.38–5.33 mIU/L). Combined with the patient's medical history, clinical manifestations, and auxiliary examinations, the diagnosis is (1) Ocular myasthenia gravis, (2) Thyroid-related eye disease, (3) Graves' disease. After discharge, the patient's symptoms gradually improved with oral bromocriptine combined with a small dose of corticosteroids. Four months after treatment,

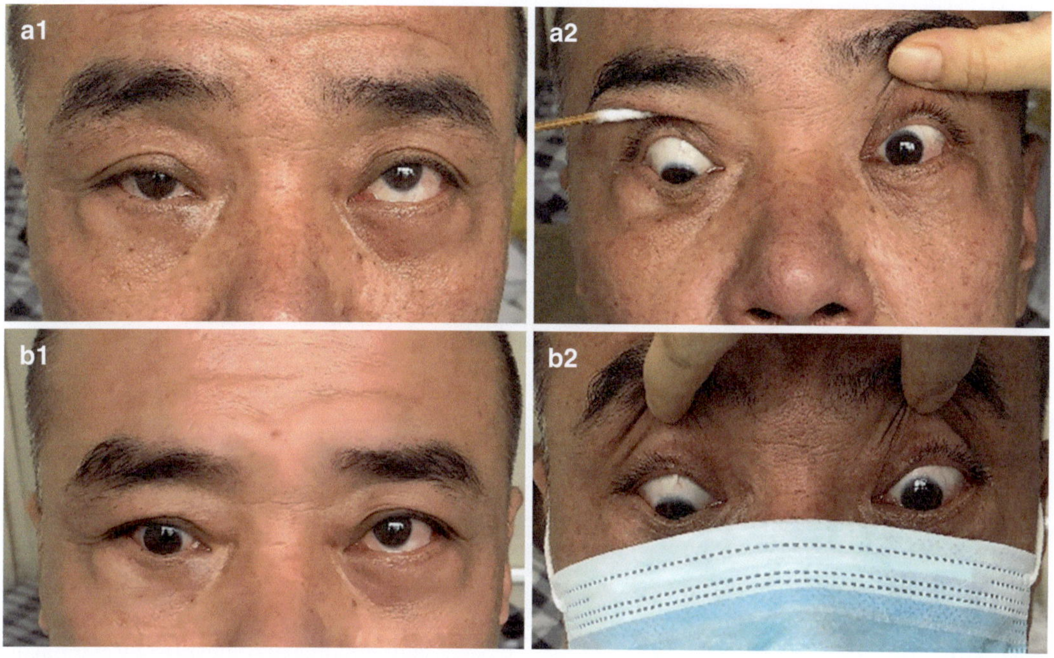

Fig. 14.6 Comparison of the patient with ptosis and left eye hypertropia before and after the Neostigmine test
Before the Neostigmine test: A1. Both eyelids droop, with the left eye deviating upward by about 35°; A2. The left eye's downward rotation is limited to −4
After the Neostigmine test: B1. The ptosis of both eyes and hypertropia in the left eye have significantly improved; B2. The downward rotation of the left eye is turning down a little bit

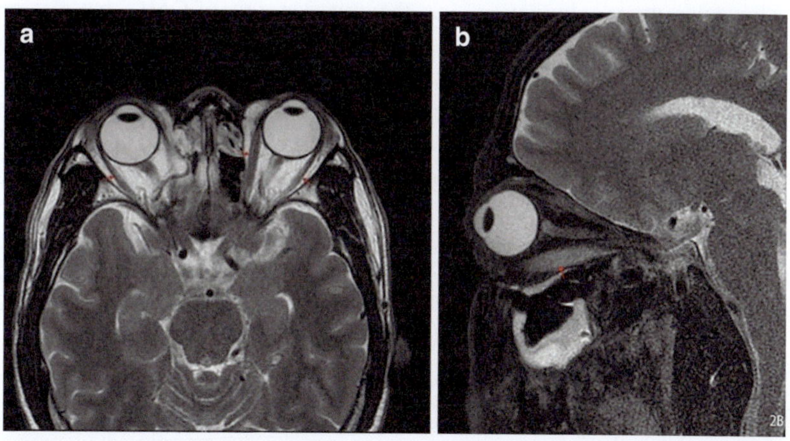

Fig. 14.7 Orbital MRI image. (**a**) Image shows thickening of the left eye's medial rectus, lateral rectus, the right eye's lateral rectus. (**b**) Image shows thickening of the left eye's inferior rectus

the eye position was normal, the eyeball downward rotation was normal, and diplopia disappeared (Fig. 14.8).

[Case Analysis]

Thyroid-associated ophthalmopathy (TAO) and ocular myasthenia gravis (OMG) are both autoimmune diseases mediated by autoantibodies. TAO is a typical eye disease associated with Graves' disease, with 70–75% of TAO coexisting with Graves' disease, characterized by limited eye movement and thickening of the extraocular muscles [9]. TAO often coexists with other autoimmune diseases, with the prevalence of coexisting myasthenia gravis (MG) being about 0.1% [9]. Myasthenia gravis (MG) is an autoimmune disease

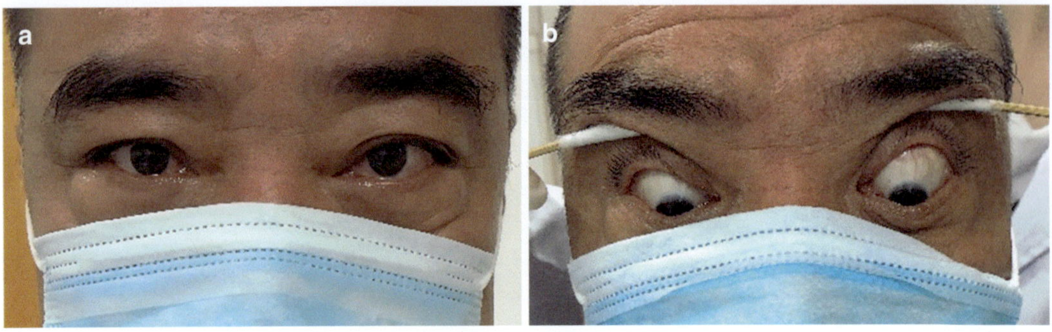

Fig. 14.8 Eye position chart of the patient with ptosis and the left eye hypertropia after 4 months of treatment. (**a**) The ptosis of both eyes has significantly improved and both eyes are in normal position. (**b**) The downward rotation of the left eye is normal

targeting the neuromuscular junction, with the most common target being the acetylcholine receptor [10]. When the symptoms of MG patients are limited to the eye muscles, it is called TAO, characterized by fluctuating and fatigable ptosis and diplopia [10]. The reasons for the simultaneous occurrence of OMG and TAO may be multifaceted, possibly due to a common genetic background and immune cross-reactions against common autoimmune targets in the eye muscles [11].

Both TAO and OMG have manifestations of extraocular muscle limitation, but the muscles involved are different. Studies have found that 40% of TAO patients have manifestations of extraocular muscle limitation, most commonly involving the inferior rectus and medial rectus, causing 5–17% of patients to have symptoms of diplopia [12, 13]. TAO causes restrictive eye movement disorders due to muscle fibrosis, so the direction of restricted eye movement is the same as the action direction of the affected muscle, often causing the affected eye to have esotropia and hypotropia, while exotropia is extremely rare [14]. Unlike TAO, OMG can involve any extraocular muscle, often involving the inferior oblique, superior rectus, and lateral rectus [2, 3, 15]. OMG causes paralytic eye movement disorders due to neuromuscular junction signal transmission disorders, and the direction of restricted eye movement is opposite to the action direction of the affected muscle [16]. The left eye hypertropia and limited downward movement of the left eye in this case do not match the results of the orbital MRI showing thickening of the left inferior rectus muscle belly.

The distinguishing points between OMG and TAO are the fluctuating and fatigable ptosis and diplopia. A review of the literature found that cases of TAO, Graves' disease combined with OMG are very rare, and the reported cases often present with diplopia accompanied by significant ptosis as the main complaint upon admission [17]. In this case, the patient's bilateral ptosis and left eye hypertropia showed a morning light and evening heavy performance, showing significant fluctuations. Fluctuation is not only a characteristic of OMG, but also an important reason for its misdiagnosis and missed diagnosis, which seriously affects the patient's quality of life and even causes disability.

When TAO and OMG coexist, young ophthalmologists with insufficient clinical experience are likely to overlook the diagnosis of OMG, leading to missed or misdiagnosed. The main reasons for missed or misdiagnosed OMG are (1) TAO and OMG have many overlapping clinical symptoms, such as diplopia, restricted eye movement, ptosis; (2) Young clinical ophthalmologists are not proficient in the mechanism of extraocular muscle involvement in TAO and OMG; (3) Not focusing on the patient's fluctuating and fatigable eye symptoms. Missed or misdiagnosed can cause patients to miss the opportunity for appropriate treatment, so that the eye symptoms do not improve, which seriously affects the patient's quality of life and even causes disability. The lesson to be learned from this case is that when TAO patients have hypertropia and limited downward movement or fluctuating eye symptoms, they should carefully evaluate OMG and promptly carry out OMG-related examinations.

References

1. Von Noorden GK. Binocular vision and ocular motility. 6th ed. St Louis: Mosby; 2002. p. 442.
2. Cleary M, Williams GJ, Metcalfe RA. The pattern of extra-ocular muscle involvement in ocular myasthenia. Strabismus. 2008;16(1):11–8. https://doi.org/10.1080/15569520701830992.
3. Akan O, Baysal-Kirac L. Ophthalmologic manifestations in myasthenia gravis: presentation and prognosis. Acta Neurol Belg. 2021; https://doi.org/10.1007/s13760-020-01556-3.
4. Trouth AJ, Dabi A, Solieman N, et al. Myasthenia gravis: a review. Autoimmune Dis. 2012;2012:874680. https://doi.org/10.1155/2012/874680.
5. Chiang LM, Darras BT, Kang PB. Juvenile myasthenia gravis. Muscle Nerve. 2009;39(4):423–31. https://doi.org/10.1002/mus.21195.
6. Huang X, Li Y, Feng H, et al. Clinical characteristics of juvenile myasthenia gravis in southern China. Front Neurol. 2018;9:77. https://doi.org/10.3389/fneur.2018.00077.
7. Fisher K, Shah V. Pediatric ocular myasthenia gravis. Curr Treat Options Neurol. 2019;21(10):46. https://doi.org/10.1007/s11940-019-0593-y.
8. Smith SV, Lee AG. Update on ocular myasthenia gravis. Neurol Clin. 2017;35(1):115–23. https://doi.org/10.1016/j.ncl.2016.08.008.
9. Davies TF, Andersen S, Latif R, et al. Graves' Dis Nat Rev Dis Primers. 2020;6(1):52. https://doi.org/10.1038/s41572-020-0184-y.
10. Gilhus N, Tzartos S, Evoli A, et al. Myasthenia gravis. Nat Rev Dis Primers. 2019;5(1):30. https://doi.org/10.1038/s41572-019-0079-y.
11. Yang HW, Wang YX, Bao J, et al. Correlation of HLA-DQ and TNF-α gene polymorphisms with ocular myasthenia gravis combined with thyroid-associated ophthalmopathy. Biosci Rep. 2017;37(2) https://doi.org/10.1042/bsr20160440.
12. Smith TJ, Hegedüs L. Graves' disease. N Engl J Med. 2016;375(16):1552–65.
13. Bojikian KD, Francis CE. Thyroid eye disease and myasthenia gravis. Int Ophthalmol Clin. 2019;59(3):113–24. https://doi.org/10.1097/IIO.0000000000000277.
14. Vargas ME, Warren FA, Kupersmith MJ. Exotropia as a sign of myasthenia gravis in dysthyroid ophthalmopathy. Br J Ophthalmol. 1993;77(12):822–3.
15. Almog Y, Ben-David M, Nemet AY. Inferior oblique muscle paresis as a sign of myasthenia gravis. J Clin Neurosci. 2016;25:50–3. https://doi.org/10.1016/j.jocn.2015.08.026.
16. Weinberg D, Lesser R, Vollmer T. Ocular myasthenia: a protean disorder. Surv Ophthalmol. 1994;39(3):169–210. https://doi.org/10.1016/0039-6257(94)90194-5.
17. Ma R, Cheng Y, Gan L, et al. Histopathologic study of extraocular muscles in thyroid-associated ophthalmopathy coexisting with ocular myasthenia gravis: a case report. BMC Ophthalmol. 2020;20(1):166. https://doi.org/10.1186/s12886-020-01431-y.

15 Typical Cases of Ocular Myasthenia Gravis

This section lists common clinical manifestations of ocular myasthenia gravis, covering pediatric ocular myasthenia gravis (<18 years old), early-onset ocular myasthenia gravis (≤50 years old), and late-onset ocular myasthenia gravis (>50 years old), for clinical doctors to refer to, in order to reduce the misdiagnosis and missed diagnosis rate of ocular myasthenia gravis.

15.1 Case 1: Pediatric Ocular Myasthenia Gravis (Ptosis of One Eye)

The patient, a 6-year-old boy, came to the clinic because of incomplete bilateral eyelid closure for 6 years.

[Clinical Manifestation] The patient, a child, started experiencing incomplete bilateral eyelid closure without any obvious cause since birth, showing a characteristic of being lighter in the morning and heavier in the evening, and worsening when tired.

[Ophthalmic Examination] Incomplete bilateral eyelid closure (Fig. 15.1a)

[Auxiliary Examination] Ice pack test positive (Fig. 15.1b), AChR-Ab(+) :3.17 nmol/L.

[Treatment] Administer Pyridostigmine 30 mg orally, three times a day. After treatment for 3 months, incomplete bilateral eyelid closure improvement (Fig. 15.2).

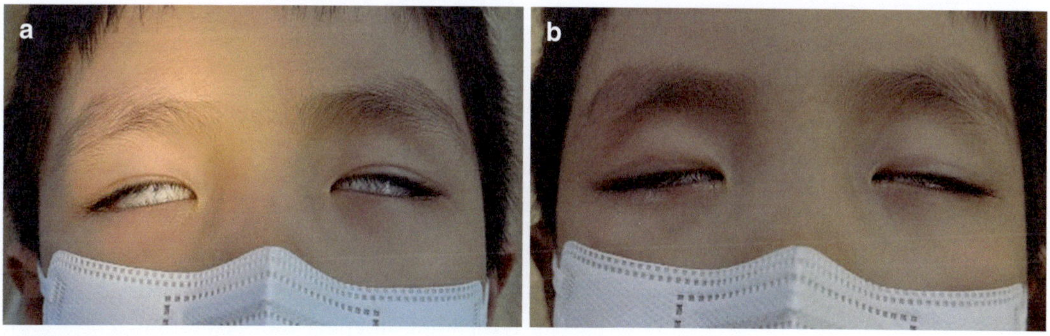

Fig. 15.1 Comparison of ice pack test in a patient with incomplete bilateral eyelid closure. (**a**) Before the ice pack test, significantly incomplete bilateral eyelid closure. (**b**) After the ice pack test, significant improvement in incomplete bilateral eyelid closure

Q. Zhou, J. Chen, *Ocular Myasthenia Gravis*, Experts' Perspectives on Medical Advances,
https://doi.org/10.1007/978-981-96-1245-1_15

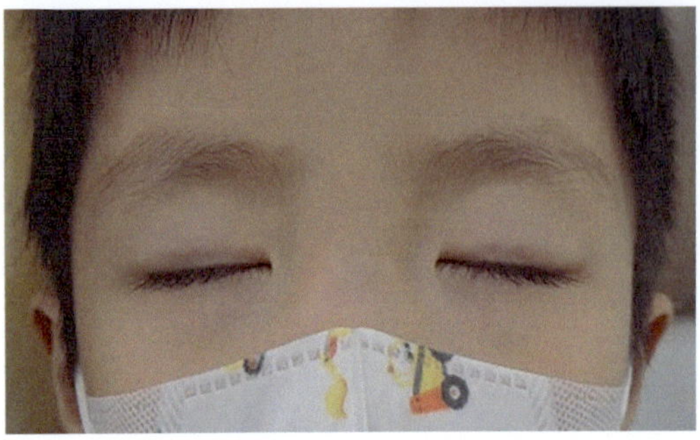

Fig. 15.2 Degree of incomplete bilateral eyelid closure after a week of treatment
After treatment, incomplete bilateral eyelid closure incomplete improvement

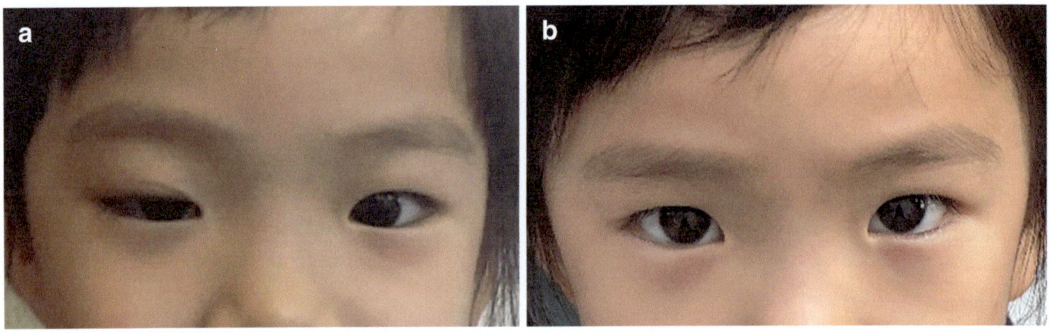

Fig. 15.3 Comparison of OMG patient before and after treatment for the degree of the ptosis in the right eye. (**a**) Before treatment, moderate ptosis in the right eye before initial treatment. (**b**) After treatment, relief of ptosis in the right eye after initial treatment

15.2 Case 2: Pediatric Ocular Myasthenia Gravis (Alternating Ptosis of Both Eyes)

The patient, a 3-year-old girl, came for consultation due to ptosis in the right eye for 3 months.

[Clinical Manifestation] The patient started experiencing ptosis in the right eye without any obvious cause 3 months ago, showing a characteristic of being lighter in the morning and heavier in the evening, and worsening when tired.

[Ophthalmic Examination] Moderate ptosis of the right eye, covering the upper edge of the pupil (Fig. 15.3a).

[Auxiliary Examination] Neostigmine test positive.

[Diagnosis] Childhood ocular myasthenia gravis.

[Treatment Course] Administer Pyridostigmine 30 mg orally, three times a day, combined with traditional Chinese medicine treatment. After treatment, the symptoms of ptosis in the right eye disappeared (Fig. 15.3b). The patient stopped medication on her own after 1 year of treatment, and ptosis in the left eye appeared 1 year after stopping the medication (Fig. 15.4). After retreatment, the symptoms of ptosis in the left eye disappeared (Fig. 15.5).

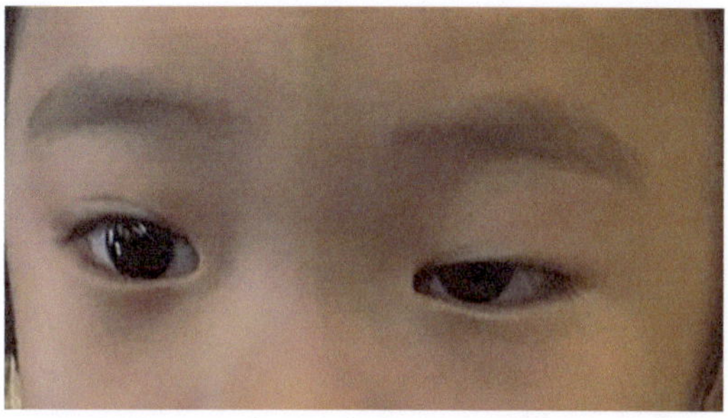

Fig. 15.4 The degree of the left eye's ptosis
Mild ptosis in the left eye after OMG patient stopped medication

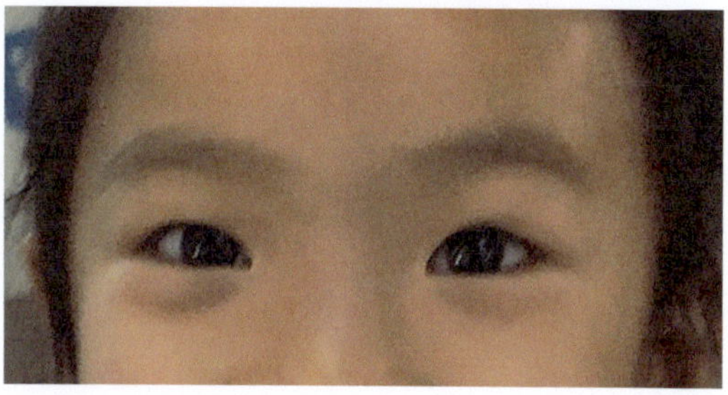

Fig. 15.5 Degree of ptosis in the eyelids after retreatment
After retreatment, relief of ptosis in the left eye

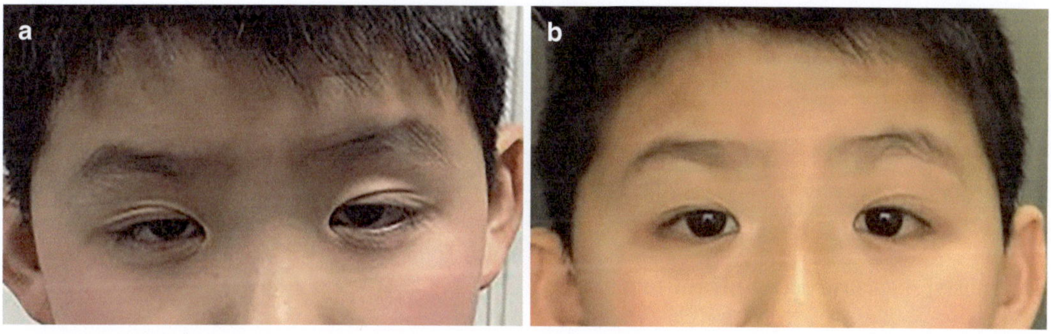

Fig. 15.6 Comparison of ptosis in both eyes before and after the Neostigmine test. (**a**) Before the Neostigmine test, mild ptosis in both eyes. (**b**) After the Neostigmine test, significant improvement in ptosis in both eyes

15.3 Case 3: Pediatric Ocular Myasthenia Gravis (Bilateral Ptosis)

The patient, a 6-year-old boy, came for consultation due to red eyes and frequent blinking for half a year.

[Clinical Manifestation] The child patient started experiencing redness in both eyes accompanied by frequent blinking without any obvious cause half a year ago. The external hospital diagnosed it as "conjunctivitis in both eyes, dry eye syndrome," and symptomatic treatment was given. However, no significant improvement was observed after half a year, so the patient came to our hospital's ophthalmology outpatient clinic for treatment.

[Ophthalmic Examination] Mild ptosis in both eyes (Fig. 15.6a).

[Auxiliary Examination] Positive neostigmine test (Fig. 15.6b).

[Diagnosis] Pediatric ocular myasthenia gravis.

[Treatment] Administered 30 mg of pyridostigmine bromide orally, three times a day.

15.4 Case 4: Pediatric Ocular Myasthenia Gravis (Esotropia)

The patient, a 5-year-old boy, came for consultation due to alternating esotropia in both eyes for 2 years.

[Clinical Manifestation] The child developed alternating esotropia in both eyes without any obvious cause 2 years ago, which gradually worsened, with significant fluctuations.

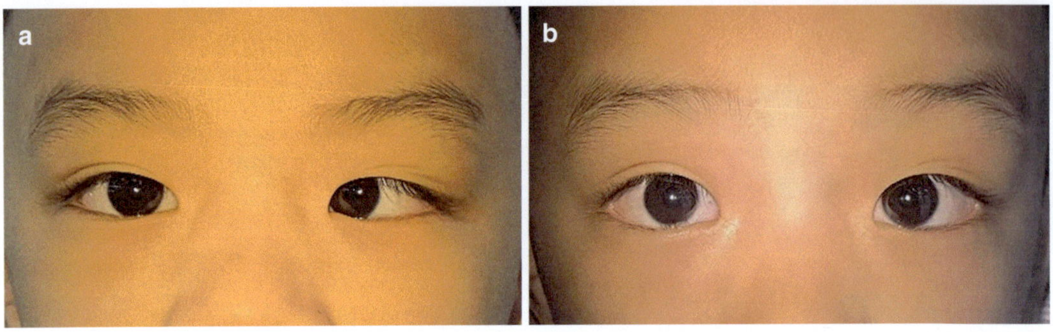

Fig. 15.7 Comparison of eye position before and after the Neostigmine test. (**a**) Before the Neostigmine test, the left eye showed about 15° of esotropia in the left eye. (**b**) After the Neostigmine test, the esotropia in the left eye significantly improved

[Ophthalmic Examination] Hirschberg test: the left eye showed about 15° of esotropia (Fig. 15.7a).

[Auxiliary Examination] Neostigmine test (+) (Fig. 15.7b).

[Diagnosis] Pediatric ocular myasthenia gravis.

[Treatment] Administered 30 mg of pyridostigmine bromide orally, three times a day.

15.5 Case 5: Pediatric Ocular Myasthenia Gravis (Hypertropia)

The patient, a 3-year-old boy, came for treatment due to progressive right eye hypertropia over 1 year.

[Clinical Manifestation] The patient started experiencing right eye hypertropia without any obvious cause a year ago, which progressively worsened.

[Ophthalmic Examination] Hirschberg test: the right eye is about 35° hypertropia (Fig. 15.8a).

[Auxiliary Examination] Positive Neostigmine test.

[Diagnosis] Pediatric ocular myasthenia gravis.

[Treatment] Administered 30 mg of pyridostigmine bromide orally, three times a day. After half a year of treatment, the eye position of both eyes was normal (Fig. 15.8b).

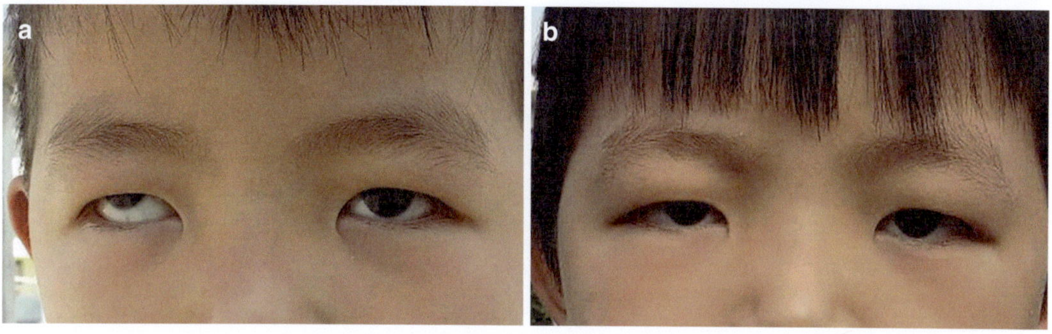

Fig. 15.8 Comparison of eye position before and after treatment with pyridostigmine bromide. (**a**) Before treatment, right eye hypertropia about 35°. (**b**) After treatment, the position of both eyes is normal after 6 months of treatment

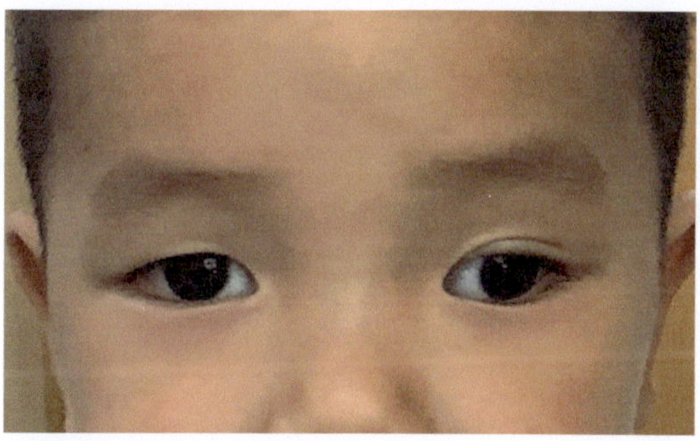

Fig. 15.9 Both eyes position before treatment
The left eye showed about 35° of exotropia and hypotropia before treatment

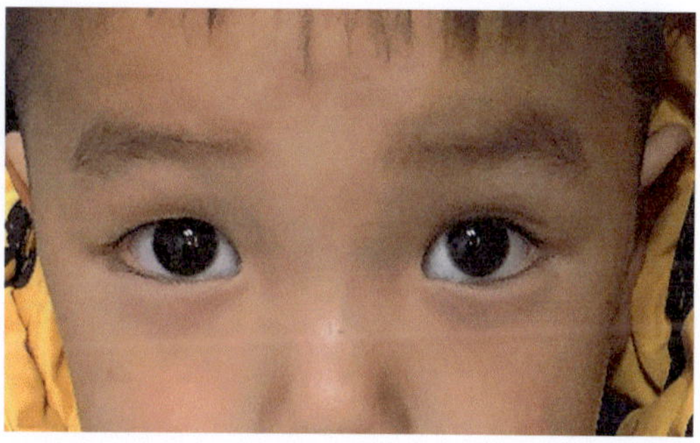

Fig. 15.10 Both eyes position after treatment
Two years after treatment, the exotropia and hypotropia in the left eye significantly improved

15.6 Case 6: Pediatric Ocular Myasthenia Gravis (Hypotropia Causing Severe Amblyopia)

The patient, a 1-year-old boy, came for consultation due to exotropia and hypotropia in his left eye for 2 months.

[Clinical Manifestation] The child developed exotropia and hypotropia in his left eye without any obvious cause 2 months ago, which gradually worsened, with significant fluctuations.

[Ophthalmic Examination] Hirschberg test: the left eye showed about 35° of exotropia and hypotropia (Fig. 15.9).

[Auxiliary Examination] Neostigmine test (+).

[Diagnosis] Pediatric ocular myasthenia gravis.

[Treatment] The child was given oral pyridostigmine bromide 30 mg, three times a day, combined with one tablet of hormone after breakfast each day. After 2 years of treatment, the exotropia and hypotropia in the left eye significantly improved (Fig. 15.10). At the age of 3, a vision test revealed severe amblyopia in the left eye with a vision of +1.0logMAR. After comprehensive amblyopia treatment (Fig. 15.11) for 3 months, the vision improved to +0.3 logMAR. After 6 months of amblyopia treatment, the vision improved to +0.1 logMAR.

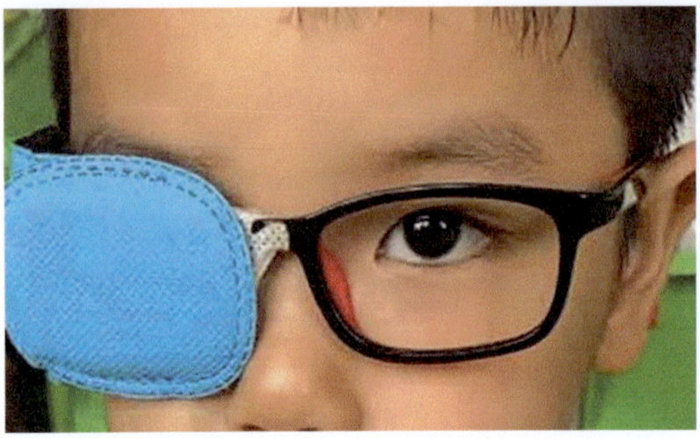

Fig. 15.11 Occlusion therapy of right eye
After 6 months of amblyopia treatment, the vision improved to +0.1 logMAR

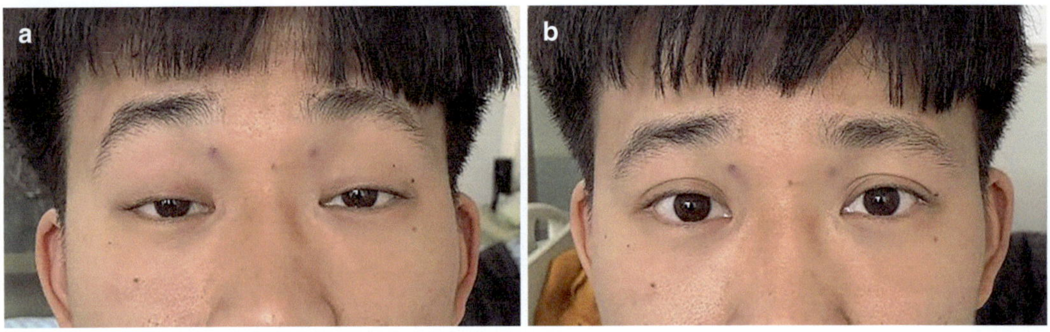

Fig. 15.12 Comparison of the patient with bilateral ptosis before and after Neostigmine test. (**a**) Before the Neostigmine test, moderate bilateral ptosis, covering half of the pupil. (**b**) After the Neostigmine test, the bilateral ptosis significantly improved

15.7 Case 7: Early-Onset Ocular Myasthenia Gravis (Bilateral Ptosis)

The patient, a young man, came for consultation due to bilateral ptosis for 6 months.

[Clinical Manifestation] The patient developed bilateral ptosis without any obvious cause 6 months ago, which was characterized by being lighter in the morning and heavier in the evening, and worsened with fatigue, with significant fluctuations.

[Ophthalmic Examination] Moderate bilateral ptosis, covering half of the pupils (Fig. 15.12a).

[Auxiliary Examination] Neostigmine test (+) (Fig. 15.12b).

[Diagnosis] Early-onset ocular myasthenia gravis.

[Treatment] The patient was given oral pyridostigmine bromide 60 mg, three times a day.

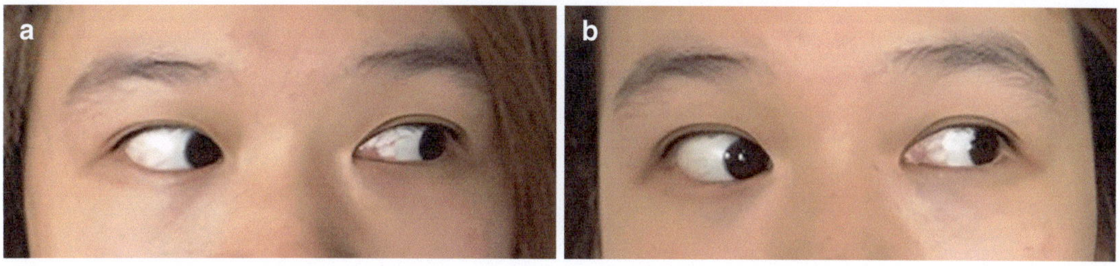

Fig. 15.13 Comparison of the right eye's inward rotation in the morning and in the afternoon. (**a**) In the morning, the right eye's inward rotation is normal. (**b**) In the afternoon, the right eye's inward rotation is limited to −1

15.8 Case 8: Early-Onset Ocular Myasthenia Gravis (Medial Rectus Palsy)

The patient is a young woman who sought medical attention for diplopia in her left eye that had been present for 3 months.

[Clinical Presentation] The patient started experiencing diplopia in her left eye without any obvious cause 3 months ago. The symptoms are lighter in the morning and heavier in the evening, and they worsen with fatigue, showing significant fluctuations.

[Ophthalmic Examination] Diplopia test: horizontal diplopia, with the largest diplopia image in the left gaze, and the peripheral image is of the right eye. The right eye's inward rotation is limited and shows a lighter in the morning and heavier in the evening characteristic. In the morning, the right eye's inward rotation is not significantly limited (Fig. 15.13a), and in the afternoon, the right eye's inward rotation is limited to −1 (Fig. 15.13b).

[Auxiliary Examination] Positive neostigmine test.

[Diagnosis] Early-onset ocular myasthenia gravis.

[Treatment] Administered 60 mg of Pyridostigmine orally, three times a day.

15.9 Case 9: Early-Onset Ocular Myasthenia Gravis (Esotropia)

The patient is a young woman who sought medical attention for left eye esotropia that had been present for 6 months.

[Clinical Presentation] The patient started experiencing left eye esotropia without any obvious cause 6 months ago. The symptoms are lighter in the morning and heavier in the evening, and they worsen with fatigue.

[Ophthalmic Examination] Hirschberg test: left eye esotropia of about 20° (Fig. 15.14a).

[Auxiliary Examination] Positive Neostigmine test

[Diagnosis] Early-onset ocular myasthenia gravis.

[Treatment] Administered 60 mg of Pyridostigmine orally, three times a day. After treatment, the left eye esotropia significantly improved (Fig. 15.14b).

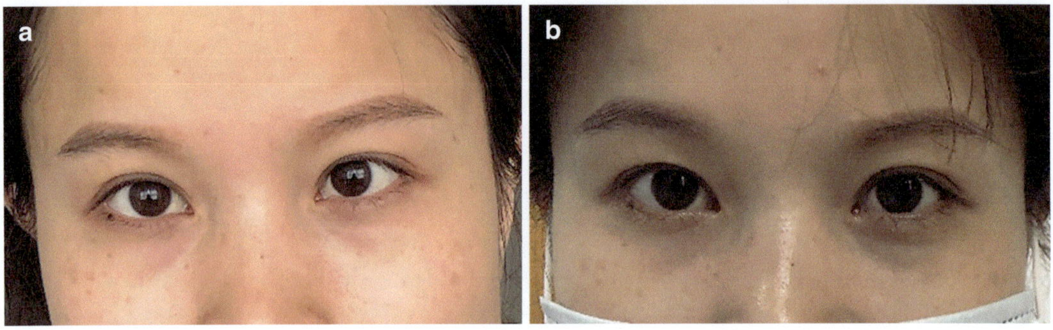

Fig. 15.14 Comparison of eye position before and after treatment in a patient with esotropia. (**a**) Before treatment, left eye esotropia of about 15°. (**b**) After treatment, significant improvement in left eye esotropia

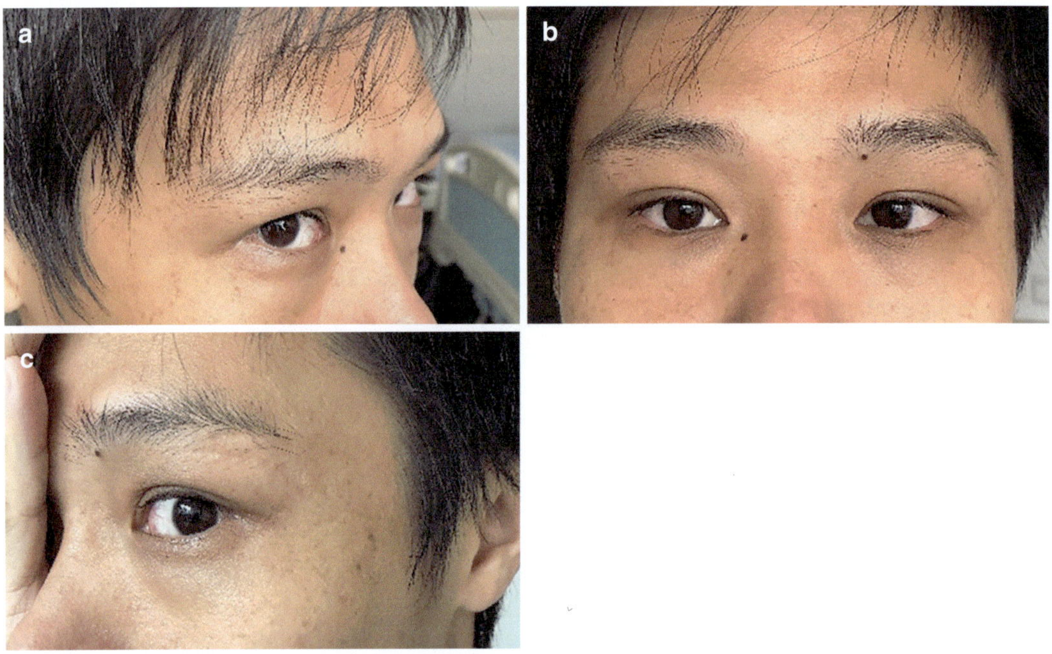

Fig. 15.15 Eye position of an OMG patient with esotropia. (**a**) Right eye external rotation limited −1. (**b**) Left eye esotropia approximately 20°. (**c**) Left eye external rotation limited −1

15.10 Case 10: Early-Onset Ocular Myasthenia Gravis (Lateral Rectus Palsy)

The patient is a young man who sought medical attention for left eye esotropia accompanied by diplopia that had been present for 3 months.

[Clinical Presentation] The patient started experiencing left eye esotropia accompanied by horizontal diplopia without any obvious cause 3 months ago. The symptoms are lighter in the morning and heavier in the evening, and they worsen with fatigue, showing significant fluctuations. Both eyes have a −1 limitation in outward rotation.

[Ophthalmic Examination] Hirschberg test: left eye esotropia of about 20°. Both eyes have a −1 limitation in outward rotation. (Fig. 15.15)

[Auxiliary Examination] Positive Neostigmine test.

[Diagnosis] Early-onset ocular myasthenia gravis.

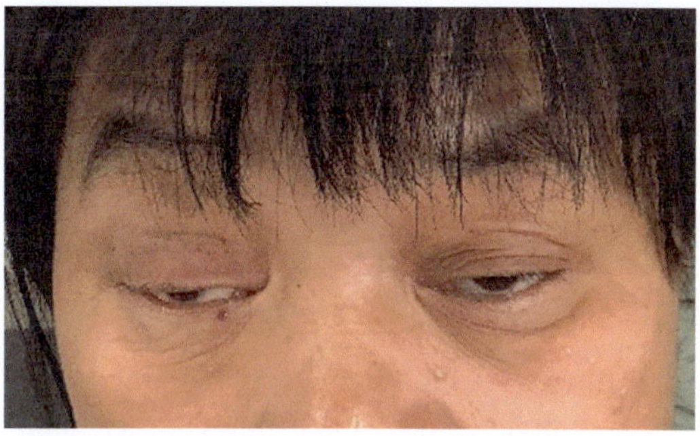

Fig. 15.16 Degree of ptosis in both eyes and alignment status
Severe ptosis in both eyes, complete restriction of eye movement, both eyes completely fixed

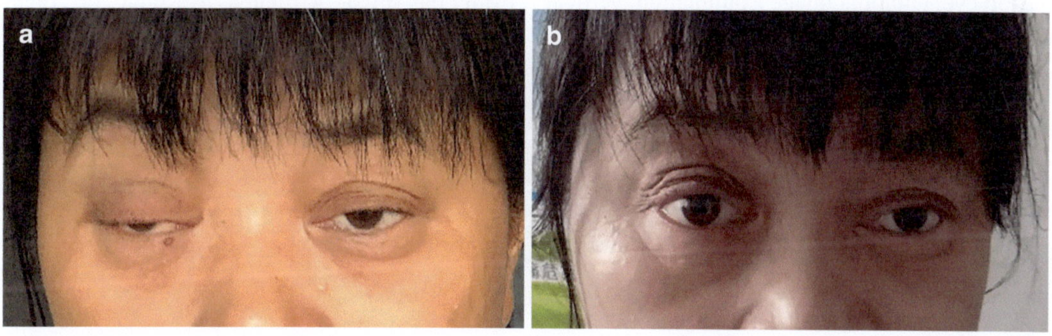

Fig. 15.17 Comparison of the patient with bilateral ptosis before and after the Neostigmine test. (**a**) Before the Neostigmine test, ptosis in both eyes. (**b**) After the Neostigmine test, significant improvement in ptosis in both eyes

[Treatment] Administer 60 mg of Pyridostigmine orally, three times a day.

15.11 Case 11: Early-Onset Ocular Myasthenia Gravis (Ptosis with Fixed Eyeball)

[Clinical Manifestation] The patient is a middle-aged woman, with progressive ptosis in both eyes accompanied by limited eye movement to complete fixation for 20 years.

[Ophthalmic Examination] Severe ptosis in both eyes, covering more than half of the cornea. Eye movement in all directions is limited −4 (Fig. 15.16).

[Auxiliary Examination] Positive Neostigmine test (Fig. 15.17).

[Diagnosis] Early-onset ocular myasthenia gravis.

[Treatment] Administer 60 mg of Pyridostigmine orally, three times a day; combined with 30 mg of Prednisone acetate, taken after breakfast, gradually reducing the dose.

15.12 Case 12: Late-Onset Ocular Myasthenia Gravis (Ptosis with Diplopia)

The patient is a 63-year-old male, who came for consultation due to diplopia for 2 months and ptosis in the left eye for 1 day.

[Clinical Manifestation] The patient developed diplopia in both eyes without any obvious cause 2 months ago, accompanied by moderate ptosis in the left eye for 1 day.

[Ophthalmic Examination] Moderate ptosis in the left eye. Diplopia image examination: vertical diplopia.

[Auxiliary Examination] Positive Neostigmine test (Fig. 15.18), positive low-frequency repetitive nerve stimulation: positive fatigue test for the left levator palpebrae superioris muscle.

[Diagnosis] Late-onset ocular myasthenia gravis.

[Treatment] Administer 60 mg of Pyridostigmine orally, three times a day; combined with 30 mg of Prednisone acetate, taken after breakfast, gradually reducing the dose.

All photographs in this book were photoed by professor Qing Zhou and used with permission from the First Affiliated Hospital of Jinan University, Guangzhou, China.

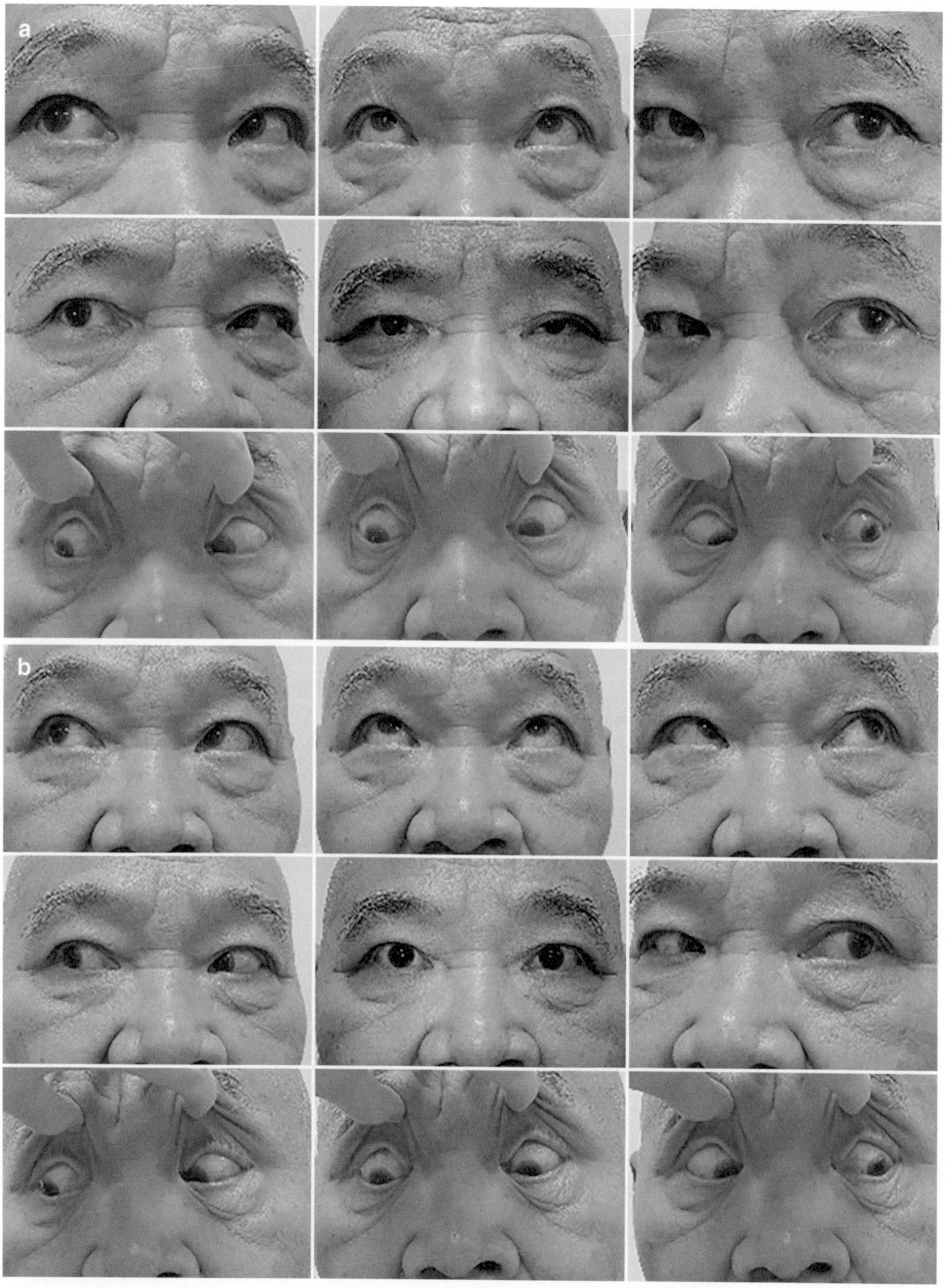

Fig. 15.18 Comparison nine positions diagram of both eyes of the patient before and after the Neostigmine test. (**a**) Before the Neostigmine test, moderate ptosis in the left eye, vertical diplopia L/R6△, the left eye's downward rotation is limited to −1. (**b**) After the Neostigmine test, ptosis of the left eye has significantly improved, and the double vision has disappeared, the left eye's downward rotation is unlimited

MIX
Papier aus verantwortungsvollen Quellen
Paper from responsible sources
FSC® C105338

If you have any concerns about our products,
you can contact us on
ProductSafety@springernature.com

In case Publisher is established outside the EU,
the EU authorized representative is:
Springer Nature Customer Service Center GmbH
Europaplatz 3, 69115 Heidelberg, Germany

Printed by Libri Plureos GmbH
in Hamburg, Germany